# The Nature of Theoretical Thinking in Nursing

**Hesook Suzie Kim, R.N., Ph.D.**

Professor
College of Nursing
University of Rhode Island

Appleton-Century-Crofts / Norwalk, Connecticut

0-8385-6652-9

83 84 85 86 87 88 / 10 9 8 7 6 5 4 3 2 1

Prentice-Hall International, Inc., London
Prentice-Hall of Australia, Pty. Ltd., Sydney
Prentice-Hall Canada, Inc.
Prentice-Hall of India Private Limited, New Delhi
Prentice-Hall of Japan, Inc., Tokyo
Prentice-Hall of Southeast Asia (Pte.) Ltd., Singapore
Whitehall Books Ltd., Wellington, New Zealand
Editora Prentice-Hall do Brasil Ltda., Rio de Janeiro

**Library of Congress Cataloging in Publication Data**

Kim, Hesook Suzie.
    The nature of theoretical thinking in nursing.

    Bibliography: p.
    Includes index.
    1. Nursing—Philosophy.   2. Thought and thinking.
I. Title.  [DNLM: 1. Models, Theoretical.  2. Nursing.
3. Philosophy, Nursing. WY 86 K49u]
RT84.5.K545   1983      610.73'01      82-16441
ISBN 0-8385-6652-9

Cover and Text design: Lynn M. Luchetti

To My Sons,
Peter and Michael,
and
To H. G. P.

# Contents

# Foreword

The increased interest of nurses in theory-based nursing is reflected in the various articles and books on the subject. The fact that so much is being written about theoretical nursing is significant because it shows that nursing is further evolving as a scientific discipline. Each publication makes a contribution in that viewpoints are set forth which can be questioned and discussed. There is something intellectually stimulating about publications which facilitate the process of reflection and debate.

This book is another on theoretical nursing. The introductory chapter highlights the *Nature of Theoretical Thinking in Nursing*. Basic terminology in theoretical thinking is presented in the second chapter which includes a general discussion on conceptual analysis. One of the unique features of the book is presentation of conceptual domains in nursing and the use of illustrations to help the reader understand theoretical analysis. Each of the domains is covered in more specific detail in three of the chapters. One chapter is used to show the nature of theoretical statements in nursing theories analysis of existing or already developed statements. It is an interesting and provocative chapter. The author's final chapter is composed of concluding remarks relative to issues in theoretical development in nursing.

Contemporary nurses will find this publication a stimulating one. They will not agree with all the points made, but they will find them provocative and challenging. Beginning students of nursing, those in advanced educational programs, as well as those practicing in different levels of nursing, will find this book a challenging one to read and discuss.

The author provides a perspective on the nature of theoretical nursing that will result in critical thinking.

Juanita W. Fleming, R.N., PH.D., F.A.A.N.

# Preface

While theoretical development in nursing has a rather short history, there are enough tensions existing within the field that call for an integrated approach to theoretical thinking in nursing. This book is intended to provide conceptual tools that can be used to delineate the world of nursing in theoretical terms. Any serious student or scholar concerned with theory building in nursing, at one time or another, would ask: "What is nursing concerned with in a theoretical sense?" It seems that for one to answer this question satisfactorily, it is necessary to have a systematic framework for the analysis of theoretical elements in the field of nursing.

I propose in this book a systematic framework that can be used to examine elements in the field of nursing and to posit important concepts in a system of order and within a boundary of specific meaning. The purpose is to understand how conceptualizations and theoretical statements are developed and refined in nursing. The primary aim of the book is to delineate theoretical elements essential to nursing, using a typology that includes three distinct theoretical domains: *client, environment,* and *nursing action.*

The book is mainly designed for graduate students in nursing who are struggling with conceptualization and theoretical analysis of nursing phenomena. My goal is to show how empirical elements in the world of nursing are translated into theoretical terms, and in turn, how theoretical concepts are specified in the real world of nursing. Specification of concept delineation is proposed within the typology. The book shows how both inductive and deductive expositions may be used in theoretical thinking in nursing. Although I discuss and analyze many conceptual and theoretical ideas expressed by nursing theorists, namely, Rogers, Roy, Johnson, Orem, and King, I do not make systematic evaluations of the values and applicabilities of their theoretical systems. I have not attempted to evaluate or criticize theories, both nursing and those from other fields of study, in a systematic or comprehensive manner. I have included in the book those appropriate aspects of nursing and other theories mainly to illustrate, expand, and apply the ideas under discussion. The purpose of the book is not to show the adequacies and inadequacies of theories for nursing as a scientific theory, but to show how such theories are similar and different in their uses of abstraction, conceptualization, and subject matter.

I focus on delineating and describing essential concepts in nursing that are thought to be important for development of theoretical systems. I contrast similarities and differences in conceptualization of nursing and elements in nursing in order to show how the same elements and phenomena are perceived differently from different perspectives, and how the same idea is concealed in many different conceptual disguises. Furthermore, the book has no specific "clinical" orientation. This reflects my bias and conviction that theoretical development in nursing should follow universally applicable conceptual strategies, regardless of the specific ways nursing problems are classified. The main emphasis is on the *how to* and the *what of* theoretical analysis in nursing.

The ideas in the book originated from my teaching of graduate nursing theory courses at the University of Rhode Island during the past several years. I owe a great deal to my graduate students who struggled with me to think clearly during those years, especially in the beginning when we did not have much written work on which to base our thinking. Many serendipitous ideas and insights were gained from working with them. I also have been most fortunate to have several colleagues at the College, especially Professors Cumings, Hirsch, and Schwartz-Barcott who are stimulating and serious theoretical thinkers. With them, I was never hesitant to grapple with even the most elementary theoretical questions. Most of all, I owe much gratitude to Professor Donna Schwartz-Barcott who has spent endless hours debating, questioning, and refining with me most of the ideas presented in the book. For granting me the most scholarly and enhancing atmosphere that any scholar would want, I am most grateful to Dean Barbara L. Tate. I believe it was this atmosphere of creative warmth that prodded me to write the book more than anything else. I am also thankful to the University of Rhode Island for granting me a sabbatical leave in 1981 so that I could devote full time to the business of writing.

As with most good things in life that need special grace, my interest in theoretical thinking received a special push from Professor Martin U. Martel of Brown University during my graduate study there. I thank him for showing me the way to question theoretically.

Even a book of this sort has to draw a great deal of support from one's personal resources. I had the most wonderful support from my children during my bout with this writing. My father and stepmother also have continued to be the staunchest supporters of my work. Among many friends who have given me much appreciated encouragements, I am most indebted to Simon for providing me early in my life the foundation for a careful self-appraisal that is needed so often, and to Kent for assuring me of the usefulness of that foundation.

My appreciation also goes to Charles Bollinger, my editor at Appleton-Century-Crofts, who gave me the kind of freedom I needed to write the book, and to Eileen Chekal who gave the most sensitive and thorough editorial assistance.

My hope is that the ideas presented in the book will create enough excitement and stimulation to propel the readers to the next stage in theoretical thinking—development and refinement of nursing theories.

Hesook Suzie Kim

# 1

# Introduction

One of the central problems in nursing theory development arises from the difficulty that the discipline is experiencing in arriving at a definition of nursing. Although we are amply supplied with many versions of rhetorical definitions of nursing, such definitions tend to establish a weak foundation for the generation of scientific knowledge, positive impact on society and the profession notwithstanding. As a matter of fact, such rhetorical definitions are the ones exactly needed as general guides for understanding what nursing is all about as a social role in the mind of the public as well as in the minds of members of the profession. In general, these definitions address social and occupational meanings of the discipline. A rigorous and exact delineation of nursing as a role and as a scientific discipline in definitional terms is necessary only when it is used as the conceptual basis for the development of a nursing theory.

Two kinds of efforts are found in the works of nursing scientists, both of which deal with the definitional ambiguities in nursing. On the one hand, several grand theorists in nursing have proposed conceptual models of an all-encompassing type. These models are used to describe: (a) what aspect or aspects of human conditions the discipline is concerned with; (b) what the members of the discipline do as the practitioners of a scientific field. Some nursing scientists, on the other hand, have focused on developing elementary theoretical statements

*The word* man *is used in the universal sense to include all of humanity. This usage does not imply sexism in any way. To use "humanity" in all instances makes some meanings awkward and unclear.*

1

that deal with a few selected concepts relevant to nursing. Although such efforts contribute to an increasingly rich body of knowledge, we must admit, albeit regretfully, that nursing as a scientific discipline is not a well-defined field yet. It is certainly true that nursing continues to be practiced in spite of the ambiguities in the definition of the role and the relative lack of specific nursing theories that guide nursing practice. This fact is important to notice as a social and epistemological reality. As Newman (1979) suggests, because of difficulties encountered in delineating nursing's subject matter, nursing theorists have become more competent in articulating what theory is rather than what nursing is.

Confusion also exists regarding what classes of phenomena should be included in a system of theoretical explanations in the nursing science. This is further confounded by the continuing debates among scholars about the differences between ''theories of nursing'' and ''theories in nursing,'' and their respective propriety, legitimacy, and relevance in the scientific study of nursing. Scientific knowledge in nursing can be expanded and enriched by studying, developing, testing, and refining *both* types of theories. This should not be viewed as a disadvantage but as an advantage for the field.

By definition, *theories in nursing* develop through the process of borrowing. Nursing as an applied scientific field has the responsibility to bring forth theories and knowledge developed in other fields. Such ''borrowed'' theories can be used to explain and predict specific phenomena with which we are confronted in our work. This involves translating and using the theories for nursing-relevant phenomena, treating them as subclasses of those for which the original theories were developed. For example, the motivation theory of learning can be applied to study patients' difficulties in learning to carry out specific self-care procedures. A modification of the theory through repeated empirical specifications in nursing situations will thus result in the motivation theory of learning in nursing. The responsibility for the selection of relevant and important ideas from such theories and for the codification into ''theories in nursing'' rests with nurse scientists. These individuals make theoretical connections between original theories and phenomena of importance to nursing, and specify the linkages, both theoretical and empirical, between them. Because nursing is concerned with several different aspects of human life, many theories from the fields of biological, social, and psychological sciences can be refined as theories in nursing.

In contrast, *theories of nursing* are those developed to explain and predict ''nursing'' as a class of phenomena proper. For such theories, it is necessary to define and differentiate nursing phenomena from the subject matter of other fields. It involves identifying the conceptual properties of selected phenomena in a specific way—that of nursing. There have been several attempts at this by such nursing theorists as Rogers, Roy, Orem, and King. Although the theoretical development in this respect is incomplete at present, there are encouraging signs for future progress. The main obstacle in this development has been our difficulty in "naming" and "describing" nursing as a distinct class of phenomena.

It is necessary to incorporate both kinds of theories into the discipline of nursing in order to aim for comprehensive understanding within the field. One must remember that the boundaries of subject matter for scientific fields, even for the well-established ones such as mathematics, chemistry, or economics, get revised through an evolutionary process. A scientific field goes through stages of boundary-definitions that are partly based on the kinds of major phenomena or subject matter it deals with, such as money flow in economics, energy and matter in physics, or personality development in psychology, and partly based on what is happening in the scientific fields in general. This idea agrees with Shapere's position (1977) regarding formation and reformation of scientific domain as constituting a unified subject matter. Well-established associations between phenomena in a scientific field are exposed to scientific scrutiny under a variety of methodologies and in entirely different perspectives. This is an ongoing process that occurs in scientific communities. Eventually, the propriety of categorizing given scientific problems into a field of scientific knowledge may be questioned, and reformulation of the boundary may occur.

The grounds used for deciding boundaries of fields may also be considered superfluous or ambiguous. Thus, subject matter may be reclassified or redescribed in different fields, especially with an emergence of new scientific fields. This happened in the nineteenth century for sociology as differentiated from economics. On this evolutionary basis, nursing as a scientific field has to go through the process of claiming certain classes of phenomena as its subject matter, and subsequently abandoning and reclaiming other subject matter as the field becomes clearer in the definition of what major scientific problems it seeks to answer. In addition, it appears that the monistic claim of a theory to be completely general and universally relevant is neither fruitful nor appropriate for nursing. Since a diversity of phenomena can be claimed as nursing's subject matter, and since the field is yet to be organized to have a definite claim to a set of specific knowledge, multiple theories are not only useful but also necessary.

With these ideas as background, I propose to show how to delineate theoretical elements for the field of nursing. My main attempt is to explain how one can examine relevant phenomena scientifically with a nursing perspective. The focus is theoretical, in that I am interested in showing the uses of theoretical tools in doing nursing studies. The emphasis is upon examining methods of theoretical delineation of those aspects of reality that require scientific attention in a frame of reference that is nursing. Nursing can claim to be a scientific field only by adhering to scientific rules of procedure, and this has to be achieved through the development of systematized theoretical statements about relevant questions in nursing.

I propose a backtracking, for I believe we are ready for a thoughtful reconsideration of what we have said about nursing in theoretical terms. We are now at a juncture after fervent discussions concerning what kinds of theories nursing should be developing, discussions that climaxed with Dickoff's and James' proposal for theories on four levels during the late 1960s. We are beginning to see the "elephant" rather than just the parts because of fertile groundwork that has gone on during the past ten years in the development of nursing theories by Rogers, Roy, Orem, Johnson, and King, among others. We are at a point in our scientific development that requires a careful reexamination of and reflection upon the construction of the theoretical domain of nursing.

To do this, a typology that includes three distinct theoretical domains of *client, environment,* and *nursing action* is proposed. This typology is suggested to classify and posit concepts and phenomena within specified boundaries. By doing this, theoretical statements can be derived or examined with a conscious knowledge of the empirical locality of concepts. This will help nurse scientists to conceptualize and theorize about observations of the nursing world, and to derive empirical explanations from theories in whatever theoretical perspective they may take. The idea is to show how empirical elements relevant to nursing study are translated into theoretical terms, and in turn, how theoretical concepts are specified in the real world of nursing. Therefore, the approach of this exposition is both inductive and deductive. This combined approach is the first step necessary for systematic thinking and an indispensable method of abstraction in developing and using theories. The "use of theories" here indicates many ways of expanding, refining, and testing that scientists do through research, critical evaluation, and theory reconstruction.

Starting with conceptualization as the first step in theory building, my intention is to begin theoretical thinking, freed from any specific theoretical bias or philosophical bent. Thus, I shall not provide formal guidelines for evaluating nursing theories, nor provide synoptic discussions and summaries of "major nursing theories."[1] Specific detail of major nursing theories and conceptual models will be analyzed and discussed in appropriate sections as examples of theoretical formulation.

In Chapter 2, the terms and concepts used in theoretical statements and theoretical analysis are defined to the extent that they are used in this book. Definitions offered for formal terms of theory construction are thought to be appropriate for theoretical thinking in nursing. The coverage on this chapter regarding definitions is far from comprehensive. There are many fine writings on this subject, and readers are referred to several original sources for understanding of terms in a variety of perspectives and uses.[2] This chapter is intended to clarify the meanings of the theoretical terms that are used throughout the book.

In Chapter 3, the rationale for the typology of three theoretical domains for nursing as *client, environment,* and *nursing action* are presented. This framework is an organizational construct, developed for systematizing many classes of phenomena that are important for nursing studies. The typology is presented here as a general guide in separating out the aspects of the real world we encounter into coherent sets of theoretical elements. It provides reference points for the analyses that follow in Chapters 4 through 6.

Chapters 4 through 6 are the main focus of the book and consider conceptualization of important phenomena at several different theoretical levels. Chapter 4 deals with the domain of client; Chapter 5 deals with the domain of environment; and Chapter 6 deals with the domain of nursing action. Concepts are delineated and analyzed with respect to their nature and scope, their empirical referents, approaches used in operationalization and quantification, and applicability in theoretical construction. For each theoretical domain, strategies for formulating the most useful and logical concepts are presented and expanded. In Chapter 4, the delineation of concepts is done according to characteristics of concepts in functional terms. In Chapter 5, the domain of environment is analyzed with respect to physical, social, and symbolic environments, and in terms of time and space. In Chapter 6, concepts are analyzed with respect to their focus either on the client-nurse dyad perspective, referred to as the *client-nurse system,* or on the nurse as actor perspective, termed the *nurse system.*

Attempts are made in Chapter 7 to show how concepts delineated within the three domains can be developed into systems of theoretical statements. Here the purpose is not to propose a theory, but rather to show what happens to an array of singular and isolated theoretical constructs when they are put into theoretical statements. Theoretical statements linking phenomena within each domain and across the domains are examined in order to indicate that relevant and critical relationships may be brought together in "theories in nursing" and in "theories of nursing."

The last chapter addresses the next step in theoretical thinking following from the exposition in this book. Some of the problem areas and issues in theory development in nursing are discussed, highlighting areas for future emphasis and concern.

## BIBLIOGRAPHY

Abell, P. *Model Building in Sociology.* New York: Schochen Books, 1971

Berger, PL. *Invitation to Sociology: A Humanistic Perspective.* Garden City, NY: Doubleday, 1963

Berger, PL and Kellner, H. *Sociology Reinterpreted.* Garden City, NY: Anchor Books, 1981

Blalock, HM, Jr. *Theory Construction: From Verbal to Mathematical Formulations.* Englewood Cliffs, NJ: Prentice-Hall, 1969

Dickoff, J, James, P, and Wiedenbach, E. Theory in a Practice Discipline: Part 1 Practice Oriented Theory. *Nurs Res* 17:415–435, 1968

Dubin, R. *Theory Building,* Revised edition. New York: The Free Press, 1978

Hardy, ME. Evaluating Nursing Theory. In *Theory Development: What, Why, How?* New York: National League for Nursing, 1978, pp 75–86

Hempel, CG. *Fundamentals of Concept Formation in Empirical Science.* Chicago: The University of Chicago Press, 1952

Kaplan, A. *The Conduct of Inquiry.* San Francisco: Chandler Publishing, 1964

Newman, MA. *Theory Development in Nursing.* Philadelphia: F.A. Davis, 1979

Nursing Theories Conference Group. *Nursing Theories: The Base for Professional Nursing Practice.* Englewood Cliffs, NJ: Prentice-Hall, 1980

Orem, DE. *Nursing: Concepts of Practice,* Second edition. New York: McGraw-Hill, 1980

Popper, KR. *The Logic of Scientific Discovery.* New York: Harper & Row, 1959

Reynolds, PD. *A Primer in Theory Construction.* Indianapolis: Bobbs-Merrill, 1971

Rogers, ME. *An Introduction to the Theoretical Basis of Nursing.* Philadelphia: F.A. Davis, 1970

Roy, SC. *Introduction to Nursing: An Adaptation Model.* Englewood Cliffs, NJ: Prentice-Hall, 1976

Roy, SC and Riehl, JP. *Conceptual Models for Nursing Practice,* Second edition. New York: Appleton-Century-Crofts, 1980

Roy, SC and Roberts, SL. *Theory Construction in Nursing: An Adaptation Model.* Englewood Cliffs, NJ: Prentice-Hall, 1981

Shapere, D. Scientific Theories and Their Domains. In F Suppe (ed.): *The Structure of Scientific Theories,* Second edition. Urbana, IL: University of Illinois Press, 1977, pp 518–579

Stevens, BJ. *Nursing Theory: Analysis, Application, Evaluation.* Boston: Little, Brown, 1979

Suppe, F (ed.). *The Structure of Scientific Theories,* Second edition. Urbana, IL: University of Illinois Press, 1977

# 2

# Terminology in
# Theoretical Thinking

## OVERVIEW

This chapter presents the definitions and meanings of the terms and concepts used in theory construction and theoretical analysis. The intention is to clarify the meanings of the theoretical terms and to provide the reader with clear definitions of them as they are used throughout this book. The meanings presented in this chapter have been taken freely from several scholars and indicate ideas and understandings of the terms that are in accordance with the accepted usages in the scientific field. The terms discussed in this chapter are: phenomenon, concept, theory, theoretical statement (i.e., proposition and hypothesis), measurement of concept, level of conceptual description and analysis in terms of holistic and particularistic modes, and method of conceptual analysis.

## PHENOMENON

The term *phenomenon* is used to designate reality, i.e., what exists in the real world.[1] Since all things and ideas exist only as mental images registered as real, a girl's love for a certain boy is as good an example of a phenomenon as an apple ripening on a tree or a patient's grimace at seeing his wound. In scientific consideration of reality, we are often, in fact almost always, exposed to multiple phenomena having similar or different meanings and characteristics. As the first

7

step in looking at reality in a reduced form, scientists must adopt a classification system by which each phenomenon is considered a member of a kind. Both the exactness of a class-definition and the scope of a class depend on the person who is categorizing, as well as on the historical conventions that have become accepted in the scientific world. By using a classification system, we are able to categorize many aspects of reality broadly or narrowly, depending upon the context in which phenomena are studied. For example, general systems theorists will categorize many different types of phenomena, such as the ecological environment of the earth, the life cycle of the butterfly, or the circuit of a computer into system/nonsystem categories. On the other hand, biologists will categorize the life forms of jellyfish, salamander, and whale into the classification system of coelenterates/arachnids/amphibians/mammals. This "naming of phenomena" into the same kinds gives order to the perceiver of reality. In fact, the phenomenon of jellyfish refers to the exact same thing as the phenomenon of coelenterates. The only difference is that the phenomenon of jellyfish is a class within the phenomenon of coelenterates. This means that as a phenomenon is thought of as having certain entities, that phenomenon is expressed as a concept. Hence, this "naming of phenomena" is concept-formation.

## CONCEPT

The term *concept* is adopted as a procedure of labeling and naming things, events, ideas, and other realities we perceive and think about. A concept is a symbolic statement describing a phenomenon or a class of phenomena. Therefore, it is expressed by a definition. While a phenomenon exists in the real world, a concept of that phenomenon is articulated in a symbolic construct, formulated through the workings of the scientist's mind. Because a concept is derived from conscious efforts to name aspects of the world, concepts may refer to a single, unique case or to a class of phenomena having the same properties that are specified in definitions. The concept of Christ, for example, refers to a single, unique entity, while the concept of crime refers to a class of deviant behaviors that violate certain legal and ethical codes of a society. Categorizing phenomena into *a class of phenomena* allows a concept to be narrow (i.e., limited) or broad (i.e., all-encompassing). Hence, pain as a concept is broader than headache, in that pain is inclusive of the phenomenon of headache.

A concept may refer to a class of abstract phenomena or that of concrete phenomena. Abstract concepts are ideas of reality and have no specific spatio-temporal referents. They refer to general cases. In contrast, concrete concepts refer to phenomena having exact references to time and space. Thus, a concept of disability, as an example of an abstract concept, may be defined as "a state in which a person is unable to carry out human actions that are normally expected," while a concept of quadriplegia of Korean War veterans is a concrete concept since it refers to a class of certain people in the world. Both abstract and concrete concepts may also take on varying levels of specificity. For example, health is a more general abstract concept than the concept of mental health, whereas fetal death in a Lying-In hospital is more general than Ann Smith's miscarriage as concrete concepts. The level of generality of viewing a given set of reality is thus a matter of choice. A conceptual ladder of abstraction, suggested as the class-subclass perspective by Blalock (1969), is a way of increasing abstractness. One can link mental images about a class of phenomena from very concrete to most general. Blalock (1969) suggests that the class-subclass perspective specifies a mode by which a generalization about a class of phenomena is made, linking more concrete subclasses to a general, highly inclusive class.

Concepts are used in theoretical statements to refer to phenomena of concern. Thus, dream is a concept in Freud's psychoanalytic theory, as are unconsciousness, id, and sleep-preservation. Rogers (1980) proposes unitary man, energy field, homeodynamics, helicy, resonancy, and complementarity as the major concepts in her theoretical model. On the other hand, Roy (1980) identifies adaptation level, adaptive mode, focal stimuli, contextual stimuli, residual stimuli, cognator, and regulator as the major concepts in her adaptation model.

Because they are constructions of the mind, concepts result from a process called *conceptualization*. Conceptualization refers to an intellectual act of delineating aspects of reality into like categories in order to give specific "names" (i.e., labels or terms). Since such delineation depends on the range of focus that is used in the intellectual act, objects of conceptualization vary in different scientific disciplines.

For our concern, the frame of reference is always nursing. This means that our interests in the real world and conceptualization of them are limited to what happens to people in need of nursing care or receiving nursing care, and how whatever happens in such situations occurs in particular ways. Thus, the phenomena of interest and concepts of them for the theoretical, scientific study in nursing are those aspects of reality that are critical to regulating nursing behaviors.

Although there are many different ways of categorizing concepts according to their characteristics,[2] for the exposition in this book I have adopted a classification scheme of *"property"* and *"process"* concepts. This classification comes very close to differentiation used by Popper (1961) and Abell (1971). Nursing is basically concerned with two kinds of reality: (a) *the state of things,* such as whether or not the patient has abdominal pain, what the anxiety level is, or what the patient knows about the emergency care of bleeding, all of which refer to the characteristics of property; and (b) *the way things happen,* such as how a person learns to take blood pressure, what a patient is experiencing when he says "I don't care," or what becomes of the digitoxin a patient takes, all of which are concerned with the nature of occurrence. The first kinds of phenomena are labeled property concepts, while the latter are considered process concepts. In this way, some phenomena may be conceptualized in both ways, property and process concepts, depending on the posture taken in conceptualization of the phenomena. For example, the concept of stress has been used by many scientists as a property concept that is expressed in terms of amount, expansiveness, or types of stress. In contrast, it also has been used by others as a process concept by which the phenomenon is identified in action terms. The course of happenings associated with the impingement of noxious stimuli on objects including humans is inclusively described in such definition. Similarly, "thought" is a property concept, while "thinking" is a process concept. As is true of any classification schema, this is also an arbitrary construct that appears to meet the test of mutual exclusiveness and exhaustiveness criteria of typology formulation.

This classification system of concepts into property and process types is useful in an analytic sense. By questioning the essense of a conceptual definition in terms of property and process, we are also questioning the focus with which conceptualization is carried out. This is theoretically important, for concepts are the main building blocks of theory. Explanations of relationships between two concepts become different according to the definitions of the concepts.

## THEORY AND THEORETICAL STATEMENT

Scientists use theories and theoretical statements as the basic tools for explaining problems of concern. Conceptualization of reality is linked into theories and theoretical statements for scientific explanations and descriptions. It has been briefly noted earlier what is meant by "theory of nursing" and "theory in nursing." At this point, it might be useful to clarify what is meant by theory and how it is used differently from related terms such as theoretical statement, proposition, and hypothesis.

_Theory_ is defined as _a set of theoretical statements_ that specify relationships between two or more classes of phenomena (and therefore, concepts) in order to understand a problem or the nature of things. The purposes of theory are multifaceted. Theory is an intellectual tool used to explain the world in which we live. The ultimate motivation, though, is in our desire to "control" the world to our benefit. Theory provides a systematic basis for sorting out regularities from irregularities. By knowing what is happening (i.e., having descriptive knowledge), and then finding out how something occurs (i.e., having explanatory knowledge), we are able to move toward knowing the kinds of changes we must make for some things to occur. While conceptualization is mainly directed toward descriptive knowledge, theory is used for explanation and prediction. As we become able to explain and predict certain phenomena, both control and prescription become possible for us. Certain phenomena can be produced by manipulating components (e.g., elements, factors, or variables) of theoretical formulations.

In practice sciences, the role of theory extends beyond simple explanation and control of phenomena. Practice sciences need prescriptions for intervention. Prescriptive theories (situation-producing theories as designated by Dickoff and James, 1968) are used to develop intervention strategies. Approaches to solving practical problems are "prescribed" according to theoretical knowledge. In nursing, Dickoff and James' classification of theories into (a) factor-isolating, (b) factor-relating, (c) situation-relating, and (d) situation-producing types has been subjected to much debate.[3] There is a general agreement, thus far, on the need for prescriptive theories, which can be applied to "regulate" nursing therapies, as the highest level of theoretical formulation in nursing.

The focus of theory is usually on unexplained phenomena considered to be problematic or important. A problem is a phenomenon that is thought to exist when connections or contrasts are made between two or more concepts, and which requires explanation and solution. For this reason, many theories are not simply drawn out of the "thin air" but are derived from other theories. Theory is a systematic way of designating orderliness between or among elements of reality. Theory is always tentative to a certain degree, since it is based on logically derived conjectures.

A good example of a theory is Freud's dream theory. He proposed as the main theoretical statements that a dream is an imagery manifestation having a latent meaning of an unconscious wish that is projected in a disguised form during sleep states, and that the dream is an indirect, substitute, and nonthreatening mode of expressing unconscious impulses in a sleep-preserving way (Strachey and Freud, 1953). Although these are rather simplified notations of his complex theory, these statements indicate the relationships he posed between the phenomena of unfulfilled wish and the phenomena of dream. Thus, dream as a variable encompasses that class of phenomena of which many different types of imageries appear and register in a person while the person is asleep. The contents of the dream Freud considers as having an important variable meaning, hence his famous work on *The Interpretation of Dreams*. Of course, it is necessary to delve further into Freud's other theoretical statements relating the unconscious and the preconscious in order to understand the main theoretical statements fully.

As can be abstracted from this example, at the most elementary level a theory consists of *concepts* and *propositions*. Propositions are statements of relationships between concepts in the theoretical system. In Freud's dream theory, two concepts are specified: dream and unfulfilled wish. The proposition indicates a causal relationship in which unfulfilled wish is postulated to cause dream. Many theoretical statements interlinked with each other make a complex theory in which several concepts are considered simultaneously in a comprehensive fashion for an explanation of phenomena.

Axiomatic theory is one type of complex theory. It follows a general format in which elementary theoretical statements (i.e., axioms) are used to derive propositions (i.e., theorems) in a theory. Axioms are theoretical statements that are assumed to be true and relate main concepts selected for a theory. Axioms are scientific laws, principles, and assumptions regarding two concepts that are taken as givens. Theorems are developed by logically interlocking axioms in a theoretical system, proposed in an effort to obtain more comprehensive understanding and explanation of phenomena in question.

Theoretical statements in a theory are merely notations that designate relationships among the conceptual elements. Theoretical statements may be descriptive or explanatory. Descriptive statements express the nature of things and characteristics of phenomena. In contrast, explanatory theoretical statements specify relationships in a causal or an associational manner among two or more concepts. Such explanatory statements are termed either propositions or hypotheses.

A *proposition* is a theoretical statement that specifies relationships among general classes of concepts. An *hypothesis,* in comparison, is a theoretical statement that is to be tested in a specific empirical situation for verification.[4] Thus, an hypothesis has a referent proposition from which it is drawn. While a proposition deals with more general classes of the phenomena in question, an hypothesis is concerned with subsets of the same classes of the phenomena. All theoretical statements have to be able to be tested or verified and should have empirical referents implied in the statements. A logical deduction is the method used to derive empirical statements from many levels of abstract theoretical statements. This indicates that concepts in propositions tend to be broader and more general than concepts in hypothesis.

An example of a theoretical statement in nursing theory would be Roy's adaptation level proposition: "The greater the adaptation level, the greater the independence in activities of daily living."[5] The concept of adaptation level, expressed as a quantitatively varying concept, is related to another concept, independence in activities of daily living, which is also expressed as a quantitatively varying concept. This statement by itself contains very little information, and a reader would not be able to understand the full meanings of the proposition. This is because the statement is derived from a theoretical system in which a special language has been developed for terms such as *adaptation level.* In this statement, whereas the concept of adaptation level is quite abstract and holistic, the concept of independence in daily living is not. The abstract and holistic concept of "independence" has been somewhat reduced to refer to certain aspects of an individual's functioning freedom, i.e., activities of daily living. By defining the exact meanings of the two concepts in the statement and specifying empirical referents of the concepts, it is possible to deduce an hypothesis of the proposition in order to test it in the empirical world.

The scope of theory is determined by the nature of phenomena it is intended to explain and the complexity of theoretical statements. Thus, subject matter for a theory may be very broad and all-inclusive or very narrow and limited. The term *grand theory* is usually used to refer to a theory that tries to handle phenomena in a general area of a scientific field, such as Parsons' general theory of action, Einstein's theory of relativity, Freud's theory of psychoanalysis, or Rogers' theory of unitary man. In most instances, grand theories require further specification and partitioning of theoretical statements for them to be empirically tested and theoretically verified. Grand theorists start their theoretical formulations at the most general level of abstraction, and it is often difficult to link these formulations to reality. In a sense, theoretical efforts for ''theories of nursing,'' such as the works by Rogers, Roy, and Johnson, seem to have focused on developing grand theories in nursing.

A more realistic and testable level of theory is what was proposed as the theories of middle range (Merton, 1957). Middle range theories in sociology such as the theory of reference group, theory of social exchange, and theory of power have been developed and tested rather successfully during the past twenty years, although many of these theories have not been integrated to form a grand theory that explains the social reality in a comprehensive manner. In nursing, very few middle range theories have been developed and tested. King's theory of goal-attainment (1981) and Riehl's interaction model (1980) may be considered middle range theories in nursing. The nursing phenomena of interest for King's theory is ''transaction'' as phenomena between the client and nurse. Transaction is used to explain the nature of goal attainment in the client.

*Micro-theory* is a term used by some scientists to refer to a set of theoretical statements, usually hypotheses, that deal with narrowly defined phenomena. Although there is a great deal of debate as to whether it should be called a ''theory,'' such a theory by itself tends to be rather limited in its explanatory power and is composed of mere postulations of hypothetical thinking. The difference among these levels of theory is not in the level of abstraction with which concepts are delineated, but in the range of explanation the theory is trying to attain. Thus, a theory can be characterized both in terms of the sophistication of its explanation and its scope.

## MEASUREMENT OF CONCEPT

Concepts are variables in theoretical statements. Therefore, it is natural to expect concepts to take some designation for measurement. This is especially necessary when scientists have to make logically sound linkages between theoretical concepts (T-concepts) and observational concepts (O-concepts). Abell (1971) uses this distinction of concepts, and it is useful when one wants to differentiate concepts in empirical studies. This is one way of distinguishing concepts used in theoretical statements and could be useful in rigorous operationalization. Abell (1971) declares that theoretical concepts must ultimately be express-ible in terms of observational concepts. The process by which scientists make such linkages is through deduction, following a hierarchy of conceptualization. This process is often referred to as the operationalization of concepts and means designations of observational concepts having immediate referents in the real world as sense impressions and as the counterparts to the theoretical concepts. A concept can take several different types of values, or character: *nominal, ordinal, interval,* and *ratio*. These are commonly accepted methods of measurement, each representing different kinds of scales of measurement (Reynolds, 1971). Regardless of the concept-type (i.e., property or process type), a concept has to be expressible in one of these quantification terms in order for it to be tested in the context of a proposition or an hypothesis.

*Nominal scale* refers to measurement of concepts characterizing the dif-ferent values a concept can take in a discrete state, such as black/red, rich/poor, dying/recovering, etc. *Ordinal scale* is based on the measure of ranking and or-dering of distinct states of a concept in a hierarchical manner so that units may be compared to one another in their rank-positions only. The difference be-tween nominal and ordinal scales may be shown by taking the concept of "health" as an example. Health measured as a nominal scale may take on such values as sick or healthy. In contrast, health measured as an ordinal unit may take on such values as highest level of health, higher level of health, moderate level of health, etc.

*Interval scale* refers to measurement of states of a concept on a constantly distributed rating rule. One position on an interval scale has the same distance from the one below and the one above. Interval scale is usually constructed in nursing research through index construction, such as empathy scale or function index. In contrast, *ratio scale* refers to measurement strategy in which a real and theoretical zero exists for the inferring of a ratio of any two members on a scale. Many scales in physical sciences are ratio scales, such as measurement for time, weight, length, etc. Scales of measurement are important so far as they provide means to align the meanings of concepts in terms of the reality.

## LEVEL OF CONCEPTUAL DESCRIPTION AND ANALYSIS: HOLISTIC AND PARTICULARISTIC MODES

The most fundamental difficulty a serious scientific thinker experiences in con-ceptualizing certain "happenings" of interest is deciding the level or the limit at which such happenings should be considered. The level of description one selects influences the kinds of theoretical questions and outcomes that are generated in the analysis of phenomena. Hofstadter (1979) treats this issue as "holism" vis-a-vis "reductionism." Holism is an analytical approach that looks at the object as a whole without paying attention to its parts. In the holistic mode, one's focus is on the generic property of object as a totality. In contrast, Hofstadter's reductionism is a mode of analysis by which the meanings of an object's parts are brought into focus. In describing these modes in a situation of listening to a Bach fugue, Hofstadter states that "the modes are these: either to follow one individual voice at a time [reductionist mode], or to listen to the total effects of all of them together, without trying to disentangle one from another [holistic mode]."[6]

The issue is this: A set of phenomena can either be viewed as a global happening or as a collection of several discrete happenings. These two approaches to viewing a set of phenomena will direct and differentiate what follows in terms of description, explanation, and measurement. For example, scientists may study humans as a whole, composed of many parts, or humans in terms of different parts. It is necessary to have a global concept of humans if one is interested in understanding humans as a totality, a unified entity. A holistic view of humans is concerned with human operations as involving the totality of the person and having meanings with respect to the total being. On the other hand, it is quite possible and sometimes desirable for scientists to study many aspects of human affairs separated out as singular or discrete occurrences without explicitly making a global reference to the wholeness of humans. Again, this is not a matter of right or wrong, but of perspective. For the exposition and analysis in this book, the terms *holistic* and *particularistic* have been adopted as two levels of description and analysis applicable to theoretical thinking in the nursing framework.

The *holistic* view of a situation or an object is directed to perceiving and conceptualizing the characteristics presented by the situation or the object as having meanings as a totality. In contrast, the *particularistic* view of a situation or an object disaggregates the situation or the object and selects out the aspects that are of particular interest for description and analysis. In a particularistic mode, the scientist takes as a given those aspects of the situation or object that exist outside of the conceptual realm of particular interest.

## METHOD OF CONCEPTUAL ANALYSIS

The first analytical technique scientists use in theoretical thinking is conceptual analysis. While conceptualization refers to the act of arriving at abstract understanding of a phenomenon, conceptual analysis refers to critical evaluation of conceptualization that has occurred. Therefore, conceptualization is an active theoretical thinking, whereas conceptual analysis is a reflexive theoretical thinking. Conceptual analysis is a critical evaluation of the product of conceptualization vis-a-vis scientific criteria of sound conceptual characteristics. In this book conceptual analysis is used as a method of evaluating the stage and rigorousness of conceptualization that has taken place regarding selected concepts.

Criteria for conceptual analysis are guidelines for examining the character-

*IMPORTANT*

istics of a concept. Reynolds (1971) proposes three desirable characteristics of scientific concepts: (a) *abstractness,* indicative of independence of time and space, allowing concepts to have more universal and general meaning-complexes that make them nontrivial and essentially important for scientific pursuits; (b) *intersubjectivity of meaning,* specifying definitional clarity and agreement among scientists with regard to phenomenal references; and (c) *operationalization and intersubjectivity of operational measurements,* indicating congruity between theoretical and operational definitions, and agreement in the methods selected to express the meanings of theoretical concepts in empirical terms. Definition of concept serves as the basic tool to indicate and reduce the meanings of abstract concepts symbolically. Kaplan (1964) also suggests that one may use either or both indicative and reductive strategies in defining conceptual terms.

The method of conceptual analysis adopted in this book uses Reynolds' criteria for scientific concepts. Conceptual analysis can be done within a specific theoretical system or without a specific orientation to a particular theoretical system. Conceptual analysis carried out within a theory is less complex since the theoretical orientation directs conceptualization toward a specific predisposition in selecting out characteristics of phenomena. Analysis of a concept without a specific reference to a theory is thus far more complex, since the concept has to be analyzed for its meaning and operationalization according to various theoretical orientations. Nevertheless, a comprehensive conceptual analysis allows progression toward theory construction as well as consequent theory analysis.

In summary, I have mainly presented my usages and understandings, omitting comprehensive discussions of various semantic, disciplinary, and scientific usages of the terms. The terms also take on somewhat different analytic meanings in the field of philosophy of science. In addition, there are many more terms and concepts used in theory development literature. A comprehensive discussion on the subject requires another kind of passion. Thus, they are not pursued here, not for a lack of passion for such a pursuit, but for the consideration of ''propriety'' of the context in which this book is written.


# BIBLIOGRAPHY

Abell, P. *Model Building in Sociology.* New York: Schochen Books, 1971

Blalock, HM, Jr. Measurement and Conceptualization Problems: The Major Obstacles to Integrating Theory and Research. *Am Sociol Rev* 44: 881–894, 1979

Blalock, HM, Jr. *Theory Construction: From Verbal to Mathematical Formulations.* Englewood Cliffs, NJ: Prentice-Hall, 1969

Blau, PM. Parameters of Social Structure. *Am Sociol Rev* 39: 615–635, 1974

Dickoff, J, James, P, and Wiedenbach, E. Theory in a Practice Discipline: Part 1 Practice Oriented Theory. *Nurs Res* 17: 415–435, 1968

Dubin, R. *Theory Building,* Revised edition. New York: The Free Press, 1978

Hofstadter, DR. *Gödel, Escher, Bach: An Eternal Golden Braid.* New York: Vintage Books, 1979

Kaplan, A. *The Conduct of Inquiry.* San Francisco: Chandler Publishing, 1964

King, IM. *A Theory for Nursing: Systems, Concepts, Process.* New York: John Wiley, 1981

Martel, MU. Academentia Praecox: The Aims, Merits, and Scope of Parsons' Multisystemic Language Rebellion (1958–1968). In H Turk and RL Simpton (eds.): *Institutions and Social Exchange.* Indianapolis: Bobbs-Merrill, 1971, pp 175–211

Merton, RK. *Social Theory and Social Structure.* New York: The Free Press, 1968

Orem, DE. *Nursing: Concepts of Practice,* Second edition. New York: McGraw-Hill, 1980

Reynolds, PD. *A Primer in Theory Construction.* Indianapolis: Bobbs-Merrill, 1971

Riehl, JP. The Riehl Interaction Model. In SC Roy and JP Riehl (eds.): *Conceptual Models for Nursing Practice,* Second edition. New York: Appleton-Century-Crofts, 1980, pp 350–356

Rogers, ME. Nursing: A Science of Unitary Man. In SC Roy and JP Riehl (eds.): *Conceptual Models for Nursing Practice,* Second edition. New York: Appleton-Century-Crofts, 1980, pp 329–337

Roy, SC and Roberts, SL. *Theory Construction in Nursing: An Adaptation Model.* Englewood Cliffs, NJ: Prentice-Hall, 1981

Stevens, BJ. *Nursing Theory: Analysis, Application, Evaluation.* Boston: Little, Brown, 1979

Strachey, J and Freud, A (eds.). *The Standard Edition of the Complete Psychological Work of Sigmund Freud,* Vol. 4. London: Hogarth, 1953

# 3

# Conceptual Domains in Nursing: A Framework for Theoretical Analysis

> Social facts cannot be adequately explained by psychological facts; psychological facts cannot be adequately explained by physiological facts; physiological facts cannot be adequately explained by chemical facts. The facts at any level of integration need to be explained and can only be fully explained in terms of that level.
>
> *William A. White*

## OVERVIEW

This chapter presents a typology of theoretical domains for nursing. The typology is composed of three domains: client, environment, and nursing action. It is an organizational construct, developed for systematizing many classes of phenomena that are essential for nursing studies. The rationale for the typology as well as the theoretical meanings of the three domains as boundary-maintaining devices are discussed. The typology is presented as a device that can help us to make sense of reality in a frame of reference that is nursing. The intellectual and theoretical preoccupation we have for understanding nursing phenomena forces us to view reality with a nursing angle of vision, and by doing this we can bring forth those elements needing critical attention to the center of the field of vision, while pushing away those with less importance and little significance into the peripheral region or to the area outside of the field of vision. The typology is

19

a tool and a guide that can be used to separate out the aspects of the real world we encounter into coherent sets of theoretical elements. In this book, the typology is used as the framework with which theoretical ideas are analyzed from the nursing perspective and as the organizing guideline for the presentation of theoretical ideas in the following chapters.

A scenario is used in the first section to show how one arrives at theoretical notions from the nursing perspective as opposed to other perspectives. The scenario is used as the basis for an examination of elements in this "reality" through the process of focusing on the nursing angle of vision. The typology of three domains is then presented, focusing on the general meanings and theoretical applicability of the domains. For each domain, examples of relevant phenomena and concepts have been delineated to show the process of conceptualization on the holistic and particularistic levels. The last section deals with the utility of the typology in conceptual development and theory construction.


## SCENARIO

Mr. Harold Smith, a 53-year-old man, sits in a bed by the window of a semiprivate room of a university-affiliated community hospital. It is six o'clock in the afternoon, and it is his third day since admission to this hospital. He appears somewhat flushed, weak, and is coughing intermittently, bringing up large amounts of brownish, mucoid sputum. He has an intravenous line in his left arm and is receiving 40% oxygen via nasal cannula. He looks haggard, seems to have some difficulty breathing, appears depressed, and is dozing on and off. His dinner tray remains on the bedside table; there is little evidence of the tray having been touched by the patient, except for the half-empty cup of tea. He has been passing liquid, greenish stools today, and feels discomfort and soreness all over the body.

His wife sits by the bed, talking little, but appearing attentive to her husband's needs and every movement. Ms. Carol Dumas, an R.N. who is the primary nurse for Mr. Smith, notices the following facts about this patient. He was admitted with a medical diagnosis of bacterial pneumonia with a question of Legionnaire's Disease. He had been diagnosed as having chronic lymphocytic leukemia seven months prior to the current admission, and was put on daily doses of chlorambucil, prednisone, and allopurinol, which apparently made him fatigued and caused abdominal discomfort. He had discontinued the drugs for a few weeks after taking them for three weeks, but had resumed taking them after a bout of flu, under the pressure of the nurse practitioner who saw him at the office for the treatment of influenza.

He had experienced three bouts of flu during the last three months, and had been treated by the physician and the nurse practitioner with erythromycin on an ambulatory-visit basis. He also has a history of chronic obstructive lung disease, associated with heavy smoking.

Ms. Dumas also noted several physical signs of significance:

1. Chest examination at admission showed rales, rhonchi, and egophony over the left anterior part of the thorax.
2. The latest readings on specimens taken on the second day of admission are:

Hematocrit ........................................................... 21%
WBC Count .......................................................... 760,000
Sputum Culture ................................................... Negative
Blood Culture ...................................................... Negative
Partial Pressure of Oxygen ......................................... 48 mmHg
Partial Pressure of Carbon Dioxide ............................. 32 mmHg
Serum pH ........................................................... 7.52

3. Latest Vital Signs

Temperature ........................................................ 39.6°C
Pulse ................................................................. 82/minute
Respiration ......................................................... 28/minute
Blood Pressure ..................................................... 106/64

4. Weight ........................................................... 162 lbs
5. Height ........................................................... 6'2"

At admission, the patient was put on cefamandole intravenously and a maintenance dose of allopurinol. In addition, erythromycin was started on the second day orally. He received two units of packed cells on the second day of admission.

He is a mailman by occupation and has been with the U.S. Postal Service since 1955. His wife works as a clerk in a small manufacturing firm. They have two sons who are married and live in the same town.

Ms. Dumas, the nurse, enters the patient's room with the IV dose of cefamandole to be put through the IV line and notices the uneaten dinner, signs of a quiet, depressed mood, and coughing. Mr. Smith's roommate is in a great deal of pain, having had abdominal surgery on the preceding day. He moans and groans aloud at times. Ms. Dumas administers the medication through the IV line and talks to Mr. Smith about his discomfort and coughing. Both Mr. and Mrs. Smith show helplessness and a degree of resignation. They appear to be very close to each other and talk about their sons and daughters-in-law in an affective manner. It appears that they are getting a great deal of support from their children, and there seems to be a sense of closeness in the family.[1]

## Appropriateness as Nursing's Subject Matter

The first question we need to address in considering and analyzing this scenario in a nursing context is to establish that there are some aspects of this reality that can be claimed to have nursing "meanings." Of course, one might say that it is superfluous to pose such a question, since the reality is occurring in a hospital to a patient, and one of nursing's important places of action is in a hospital with patients. Such obviousness notwithstanding, we shall make a formal claim upon this situation by applying the definition of nursing.

Nursing is a service to people for the promotion of individual health. Thus, a situation requiring services or interventions of health promotion is a legitimate place for nursing. Since Mr. Smith's situation requires interventions that are unique to nursing, it is justifiable for us to claim this reality as having nursing phenomena. Yet this does not mean that the situation cannot be claimed by other scientific disciplines as having unique meanings and problems that are only applicable to their fields. This possibility is the main reason for the necessity for a specific angle of vision, a selected frame of reference, in studying a given phenomenon. While nursing is concerned with health and health care, not all aspects of health and health care constitute the proper subject matter for nursing. By adopting Berger's phrase (1963), we might state that nursing does not study phenomena that another field is unaware of, but it examines and studies the same phenomena in a different way, *from the perspective of nursing.*

### Meaning in Nonnursing Perspectives

In an effort to make clear the later discussions concerning the perspective of nursing in analyzing the scenario, let us examine possible claims of phenomena in the scenario by other nonnursing perspectives first. We will look at the perspectives of medicine, pharmacology, social service, medical science, and psychology in order to contrast the meanings of studying the same reality in different ways with different angles of vision.

First, let us take the perspective of medicine. The medical frame of reference in pursuing problems of health is based on a number of carefully delineated models of normal and abnormal human conditions and of *modus operandi* for diagnosing and handling such human conditions as diseases and pathologies. In the medical frame of reference, a physician will pose the following questions related to the scenario because these or others similar to these are important aspects of the phenomena to medicine.

1. Mr. Smith's blood and sputum cultures that were performed at the time of admission and on the second day of the admission were reported with negative growth. Why were the cultures negative when it is apparent that he has inflammation in the lungs and bronchi?
2. How did the taking of immunosuppressive drugs influence the prognosis of Mr. Smith's pneumonia?
3. How did the characteristics of lung sounds and sputum change over the course of treatment?
4. Why did the patient have diarrhea while remaining febrile?
5. Should erythromycin be given orally or intravenously? How long

should the patient be on antibiotics, in the light of repeated pulmonary infections?

6. Should Mr. Smith receive a packed-cell transfusion?

These questions point out the medical frame of reference; the reality of the scenario presents itself in the phenomena of abnormal clinical findings (e.g., lung sounds, sputum, diarrhea, vital signs, blood counts, plasma oxygen, and carbon dioxide levels, etc.), confirmations of and deviations from ideal-type diagnosis, and susceptibility and/or appropriateness of medical treatments. Therefore, the medical frame of reference directs attention to studies of medical diagnosis, pathological findings, and treatment protocols necessary for removal of pathologies.

The pharmacological frame of reference will question the problems of possible interaction between cefamandole and allopurinol, the excretion rate of erythromycin in a patient with possible liver pathology, and the compatibility of erythromycin with cefamandole, however unimportant these questions may be to other scientific fields. A pharmacological orientation calls attention to drug-interactions, absorption and excretion of drugs, and drugs' effects on physiological functioning. Hence, the situation with Mr. Smith is a case in which such pharmacological questions may be raised.

In contrast, the social service frame of reference will view the reality of the scenario in terms of: (a) Does Mr. Smith have disability insurance coverage that will assure a continued income for the family? or (b) Is the family going to need some kind of assistance with social welfare services in the event of Mr. Smith's discharge from the hospital? The frame of reference for social service is in effective and efficient utilization of private and public resources in case of crisis and disruption in individual and family life. Thus, it is appropriate for this perspective to examine the reality of the scenario with such questions presented above.

These examples of questions based on different frames of reference indicate to us how the same situation may be perceived in many different ways for solutions of specific kinds. These questions can become the basis for an inductive study of phenomena, posed in the different perspectives, seeking different solutions.

Another way of linking the reality of this scenario with scientific studies is through a deductive system in which scientists identify appropriate aspects and elements of the reality as empirical counterparts to theoretical concepts they are investigating. For example, a medical scientist who is interested in relationships between immunosuppressive drug use and occurrence of infection can easily include Mr. Smith as a possible sample in such a study. In a similar way, a psychologist who is interested in studying relationships between the concepts of locus of control and decision-making may want to investigate Mr. Smith's smoking behavior in that perspective.

Different definitions of a situation made in the context of scientific angles of vision allow divergent theoretical questioning and multiple empirical conceptualizations. This is indeed what is meant by studying the same phenomenon in different ways.

### Perspective of Nursing

We now turn to the question of how nursing should then perceive the phenomena in this scenario. We can pose many questions haphazardly as the questions were presented with other perspectives in the above section. However, since the aim is to present a systematic view of this reality from the nursing perspective, I propose a method by which the phenomenal elements in the scenario are dissected and disentangled rather than conceived as a conglomerated, global phenomenon. This does not mean that the scenario cannot be perceived and conceptualized as one global phenomenon; yet, the theoretical usefulness of such an approach may be too complicated at this point, or meaningless for nursing explanations.

It is somewhat like viewing Picasso's *Les Saltimbanques (The Entertainers)*. A viewer as a lover of art appreciates the total mystery and beauty of the painting as a piece of work that moves the heart. He or she feels a certain message from the painting, such as "solitude," "pathos," or "waiting." Whatever message the viewer perceives, he or she perceives from the totality of the painting as it is presented to him or her. This is the holistic mode of perception as defined in Chapter 2. In this mode, the viewer is totally involved in the piece of art as a whole thing representing a specific meaning as a whole.

However, another viewer may attain quite a different kind of appreciation and understanding of the painting by dissecting the painting and viewing it in one of many possible different meaning-systems. These may include: (a) the physical attitudes depicted in the painting—how each person in the painting stands and looks to another; (b) the emotional tones of the painting—how the emotions are depicted by the painter in different expressions assumed by the "entertainers"; or (c) the blending of color tones—how colors are used for the personage and the background. This second viewer uses a specific guideline for viewing art (i.e., a particular mode of perception and analysis within a frame of reference that is art) in order to understand the meanings of the given phenomena. This second viewer's understandings would be specific to interrelatedness of objects on canvas, the mixture of emotional tones as depicted in images with figures and colors, or the use of color. This viewer has thus adopted the particularistic mode of perception.

In essence, the quality of impressions attained by viewers of a painting, such as the first viewer, would depend on the extensiveness and refinement of the general knowledge the viewer has acquired about painting, art, and beauty. In contrast, the second viewer adopts an analytic posture for understanding what

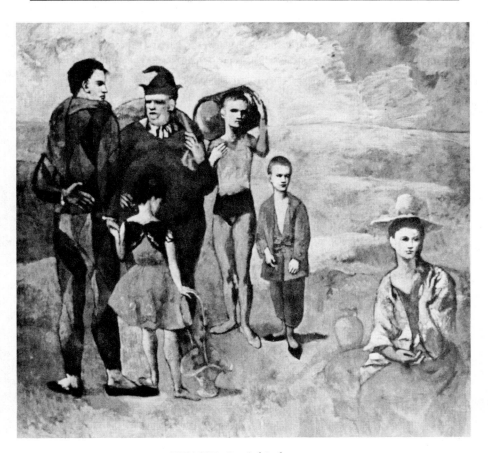

PICASSO: *Les Saltimbanques*

is presented before him or her, making it possible for the viewer to appreciate the art in the context of its selected meanings and qualities.

Thus, the proposed method here is to adopt the analytical mode of examining a phenomenon so that we may be able to understand the hidden aspects of the reality and examine various elements in a phenomenon with different frames of reference. Since this analytical method is akin to the particularistic mode of description and analysis, it is necessary to make an eventual consolidation with the holistic mode of analysis. The essential distinction between holistic and particularistic analysis is in the focus of description. Holistic analysis is aimed at examining properties and forces of an object or a situation as a whole. Particularistic analysis, on the other hand, is aimed at focusing on a specific aspect or element of a situation or an object without having an explicit regard for the whole. Therefore, for any particularistic level, there is a related holistic level, and for any holistic level there is a more global holistic level, making the first holistic level particular.

These thoughts on analytical modes indicate that it is possible to pose questions regarding the scenario from the nursing perspective on various levels. We can abstract the following elements from the scenario that are directly related to Mr. Smith, the *client:*

1. Mr. Smith is tired, anorexic, underweight, and generally uncomfortable.
2. He suffers from chronic nonreversible damage to the lungs, and is experiencing a long-term debilitation requiring continued compliance with medical treatments.
3. He has a history of self-discontinuation of drug treatment, as well as a history of resuming the treatment under professional pressure.
4. He is attached to an IV line and oxygen therapy, which limit his activities and prevent him from smoking at present.
5. His respiration is labored, he has a productive cough, and he is diarrheic.
6. He is repeatedly attacked by respiratory infection.
7. He is depressed and appears helpless.

These are major elements of the scenario requiring explanations and understanding in order for nursing to provide effective care to Mr. Smith.

We can also abstract different elements from the *environment* of Mr. Smith. The following can be specified as having significant meanings to nursing:

1. Mr. Smith is in a semiprivate room in which the roommate is suffering from acute pain. There are noises around him always.
2. His wife sits at the bedside, appearing very supportive to his needs.
3. His children live in the same town and are close to their parents.
4. The nurses on this unit are familiar with Mr. Smith, since he had been hospitalized on this unit on two previous occasions.

These are some of the elements in the environment that are relevant in gaining answers to nursing questions, e.g., do these factors influence or explain Mr. Smith's health in any way, or do any of these factors have influence on the way nursing care is provided to Mr. Smith?

In addition to these two sets of phenomenal elements in the scenario that are important to nursing's understanding of Mr. Smith's care, the following questions must be posed with specific regard to *nursing interventions:*

1. What should be Ms. Dumas' (the nurse's) response to Mr. Smith regarding the uneaten dinner, his general discomfort, and his malaise?
2. What kind of interactive approach should the nurse use with Mr. Smith? Why would one specific approach be better than others?
3. What should the nurse do in adding the medication to the IV line?
4. How could the nurse assist Mr. Smith to cope with the effects of immunosuppressive drugs and with the repeated respiratory infection?
5. What are therapies that can be carried out to ease Mr. Smith's discomfort caused by diarrhea?
6. How did the nurse organize the data on Mr. Smith?
7. What are the alternative approaches the nurse has formulated for the delivery of nursing care during Mr. Smith's hospitalization?
8. What are the plans the nurse has made for Mr. Smith regarding follow-up care and recovery?
9. How should the nurse assist Mr. and Mrs. Smith to handle the chronicity of his illness?

These questions are related to the kinds of nursing activities the nurse needs either to carry out or to consider carrying out for the patient. These are secondary to understanding obtained regarding the client and his environment.

These three sets of delineations indicate that it is possible to disentangle the situation of nursing care into three areas of focus: *the client, the environment,* and *the nursing action.* Furthermore, the questions posed in this nursing perspective are different from those raised from the other nonnursing perspectives. These are nursing questions, raised for the deeper understanding and explanation of the situation. The goal is to give nursing care to Mr. Smith that is scientifically appropriate and effective. This analysis leads us to a typology that can be used systematically to analyze elements in nursing situations: a typology of three domains—client, environment, and nursing action.

## THE TYPOLOGY—THREE DOMAINS

Three domains of client, environment, and nursing action are proposed at this point as components of a typology for conceptualization from the nursing perspective. This classification scheme is a way of disentangling realities, phenomena, and concepts within the nursing perspective. The three domains of this framework direct identification of concepts within specific phenomenal boundaries, and are suggested for use in properly "locating" phenomena of importance to nursing studies.

This suggested utility is quite different from the purposes linked to the frameworks of theory analysis advanced by Newman (1979), Hardy (1978), and Stevens (1979). These domains of the typology are somewhat similar to Stevens' commonplaces of nursing theories, which are identified as (a) nursing acts, (b) patient, (c) health, (d) relationship between nursing acts and patient, (e) relationship between nursing acts and health, and (f) relationship between patient and health (1979). However, Stevens' commonplaces are used as the basis for identifying major components of theories, especially in evaluating the comprehensiveness and focus, rather than as an aid to conceptualization of nursing phenomena.

Similarly, Yura and Torres (1975) identified four subconcepts—man, society, health, and nursing—as the most commonly identified components for theoretical formulations in nursing as articulated in baccalaureate curriculum. Also, Fawcett (1978) adopted person, environment, health, and nursing as the units specifying the phenomena of interest to nursing science and as the essential components of nursing theories. Although the proposed typology of three domains is an attempt to refine such suggestions, the major purpose of the typology is different from the motivations expressed by Torres and Yura and Fawcett. Their main interests were to identify essential concepts in nursing theories. The idea is to use the typology to identify essential aspects of nursing as contained within the three domains. This typology is a conceptual tool by which nursing scientists can identify a locus of concepts and phenomena within specific domains. Although the domains may be used to test theoretical comprehensiveness, the main purpose for the typology is in its usefulness in theoretical thinking about the scientific field of nursing.

More importantly, this typology can be used to define the nursing angle of vision in viewing the world of health care. Any conceptual or theoretical development has to have a specific reference to nursing in order for it to have value to the scientific field of nursing. The primary concern regarding theoretical thinking in nursing is not that of comprehensiveness of nursing theories, but is in ensuring that what we develop theoretically has nursing significance. As shown in the following introductory discussions regarding each domain, and in more in-depth expositions offered in Chapters 4 through 6, the domains are used to make sense of concepts and phenomena we study in nursing.

## The Domain of Client

Clients present to us rich arrays of phenomena requiring various types of considerations, understandings, and interventions, as shown in the preceding discussions regarding Mr. Smith. The domain of client is concerned with those theoretical issues that pertain only to the client. The focus is on what is happening with, presents in, or refers directly to a client. In addition, when the client is the focus, we are also only concerned with those elements in the client relevant to nursing. The ultimate reason for nursing to examine "client" as the focus is that, by understanding happenings (phenomena) in the client, nursing can: (a) gain knowledge regarding the client's problems, (b) formulate generalized notions about why problems exist, and (c) deliver the most effective and needed nursing care to the client.

The elements of the scenario that pertain to the domain of client were identified earlier. Table 1 shows how such phenomenal elements are then made to have some meaning-relations with specific concepts in the domain of client. Concepts such as fatigue, discomfort, chronicity, etc., therefore, can be examined and analyzed as theoretical concepts for explanations. Some of the concepts are holistic concepts, while others are particularistic on several different levels of abstraction. Thus, concepts in the domain of client can be delineated in both the holistic and particularistic modes.

For example, on a holistic level, a patient who walks into an emergency unit with a swollen and injured face is considered and described in terms of macroscopic factors that are *sui generis* to the human person and that describe the person as a whole, such as healthy, sick, happy, depressed, or dying. It also involves a perception of the individual with respect to characteristics that depict the person as the basic unit of analysis. Thus, the following description of the person in this holistic mode of analysis might result:

Marjorie Johnson, a woman of middle years with a slight figure, who appears fearful and nervous in her posture, has gross injuries of old and fresh contusions and lacerations on her face. Her face appears distorted and her posture is

**TABLE 1. An Illustration of Relationships between Selected Phenomena and Concepts in the Domain of Client**

| Phenomenal Elements | Concepts |
|---|---|
| Tired; anorexic; underweight; general discomfort; depressed | Fatigue Lassitude Anorexia Depression |
| Chronic nonreversible lung disease Lymphocytic leukemia | Chronic illness Chronicity |
| Intravenous infusion Oxygen therapy | Invasion of body Supplementation |
| Self-discontinuation of drug | Noncompliance |
| Labored respiration Productive cough | Respiratory distress |
| Repeated respiratory infection | Chronicity Recidivism Illness |
| Mr. Smith as a person | Man |

agitated. She looks as though in pain yet indicates that the injuries do not hurt.

On the contrary, on a particular level, this same patient is considered and described with a particular focus, the injury. A description with a particularistic focus on the injuries of Marjorie Johnson will result in the following:

Marjorie Johnson's facial injuries consist of a two-degree edema on the left side of the face, with a contusion of 2 cm diameter around the left cheekbone area, and a superficial cut in the mucosa of the upper lip that is bleeding intermittently. There are several small contusions near the forehead that are sensitive and painful to pressure.

The focus of the holistic description within the domain of client is the person as a whole, as a human person, while the focus of the particularistic description is the injury, in this instance. In the theoretical arena, both levels of description and analysis are necessary, so far as each level is selected for appropriate theoretical explanations.

A more comprehensive discussion and a detailed exposition for concepts and phenomenal elements in the domain of clients can be found in Chapter 4.

## The Domain of Environment

The second domain of attention for dissecting phenomena in nursing situation is the domain of environment. The environment of the client is thought to be composed of physical, social, and symbolic components, varying in temporal and spatial contexts. Environment refers to the external world that surrounds the client and is composed of both immediate and remote elements.

Table 2 shows the linkages between the phenomenal elements that were identified in the preceding section regarding Mr. Smith and general concepts that are thought to encompass those phenomenal elements. These phenomenal elements and concepts identified for Mr. Smith's situation have theoretical significance for nursing to the extent that (a) scientific scrutiny of such concepts will illuminate understandings and explanations regarding the client's problems, and (b) theoretical understandings of concepts and their relationships to other phenomena will influence the nursing interventions.

Just as we examined phenomena and concepts in the domain of the client in two analytic modes, so too the domain of environment also can be subjected to both modes of analysis. Environment in a holistic mode of analysis takes the form of global surrounding having multiple yet coherent influence as a whole to the client. In contrast, environment can be analyzed in a particularistic mode as composed specifically of physical, social, and symbolic parts. A more comprehensive analysis of the domain of environment is presented in Chapter 5.

**TABLE 2. An Illustration of Relationships between Selected Phenomena and Concepts in the Domain of Environment**

| Phenomenal Elements | Concepts |
| --- | --- |
| Hospitalized in a semiprivate room<br>Has a roommate who is noisy<br>Pain<br>Noise | Sensory overload<br>Territoriality<br>Social isolation |
| Presence of wife | Affection<br>Significant other<br>Dependency<br>Empathy<br>Concern |
| Wife and children | Social support<br>Affection<br>Dependency<br>Nurturance<br>Social interaction |
| Presence of nurse | Empathy<br>Nurturance<br>Dependency |

### The Domain of Nursing Action

This domain encompasses phenomena and concepts related to *what* nurses do in the "name of nursing." It includes exchange between the nurse and the client; it encompasses the nurse acting for the client; it involves the nurse acting on the client; and it also pertains to the nurse formulating, thinking about, and contemplating nursing actions. The domain includes two distinct types of theoretical elements: (a) phenomena and concepts of performing and carrying out nursing activities in the presence of the client, and (b) phenomena and concepts related to the nurse's independent activities that are concerned with making decisions, formulating plans, and setting priorities. The first type *(the client-nurse subsystem)* invariably involves the nurse in direct contact with the client, whereas the second type *(the nurse subsystem)* includes fundamentally intellectual and mental phenomena that occur in the nurse. Such concepts as touch, empathy, energy transfer, therapeutic communication, comfort measures, collaboration, and negotiation belong to the first type of this domain as concepts relevant to nursing study. For this subsystem, the main theoretical question is related to the nature of nursing intervention used for solving the client's problems and the methods of delivering interventions to the client in client-nurse dyad situations. For example, we are not only interested in what ways a nurse adopts an empathetic attitude with a given client, but we also are interested in obtaining scientific understandings of how empathy influences the client's well-being and what nurse characteristics influence the way it is used in client-nurse situations.

For the subsystem of the nurse, the main theoretical question involves the methods by which nurses make decisions regarding nursing care and what techniques are adopted for solving nursing problems. Thus, concepts such as critical nursing judgement, prioritization of nursing-care needs, and decision-making belong to this subsystem of the nursing action domain.

Table 3 shows the linkages between the questions presented regarding the nursing care of Mr. Smith in the preceding section and relevant theoretical concepts. These are examples of concepts that require theoretical understanding if nursing actions are to make scientific sense. As the examples show, some concepts of nursing actions are particularistic, such as comfort-inducing strategy and use of energy, while others are holistic, such as caring, empathy, and influence. This, then, also suggests that phenomena and concepts in the domain of nursing action can also be analyzed in both modes, holistic and particularistic. A more indepth exposition regarding the domain of nursing action is presented in Chapter 6.

In a way, the typology of three domains proposed in this section is a way of reshaping the world to fit our purpose, to identify only those critical elements for scientific and theoretical scrutiny within the nursing perspective. The three domains are not separated in any formal way, except in their boundary specifications that enable locus designations of phenomena and concepts. The ways the domains are conceptually divided for this purpose is summarized in Figure 1. The figure shows subcategories that make a conceptually meaningful sense and

### TABLE 3. An Illustration of Relationships between Selected Phenomena and Concepts in the Domain of Nursing Action

| Phenomenal Elements | Concepts |
|---|---|
| *The Client-Nurse System* | |
| Nurse's responses | Comfort-inducing strategy |
| Nurse's approach | Empathy |
| | Caring |
| IV medication | Therapeutic application |
| | Use of energy |
| Observation of patient's problems | Patient teaching |
| | Influence |
| | Collaboration |
| *The Nurse System* | |
| Organization of data | Nursing assessment |
| Formulation of alternative in nursing care | Priority setting |
| | Nursing decision-making |

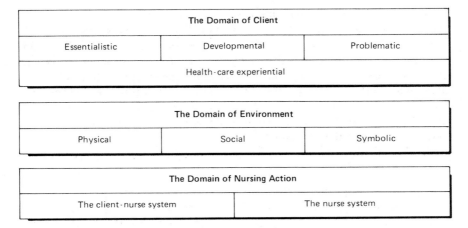

*Figure 1.* The three theoretical domains of nursing and their conceptual sub-boundaries.

analytical clarification in thinking about each domain, as discussed in this section and as also expanded in the later chapters. This typology can only serve as a way to see things more clearly and to understand the proper contexts of conceptual and theoretical development. It is a tool that can make the development of conceptual clarification less painful and less haphazard.

## UTILITY OF THE TYPOLOGY IN CONCEPTUAL DEVELOPMENT

The question, then, is how this typology aids conceptual development in nursing. The examples of the scenario and the linkages shown between the observational elements (phenomenal elements) and the theoretical concepts for the three domains as presented in Tables 1, 2, and 3 refer, in fact, to the first-level inductive conceptualization. We have defined the boundaries for understanding the phenomenal elements in reality as having specific locus of meaning with respect to client, environment, and nursing action. This process enables the inferences of realities to abstract concepts and makes the understanding of aspects of reality in a general, theoretical sense, rather than as distinct, isolated, novel situations. This disentanglement of reality into many different observational concepts within the three domains also makes scientists view reality in a detached, analytic manner.

A reverse approach of deductive conceptualization for a scientist in approaching reality is also possible within the typology. For example, a scientist who is interested in the theoretical concept of fatigue will first define the concept to refer to phenomena in the domain of client. Following this definition, the scientist will formulate observational referents of the concept. The actual observation and analysis occur as the scientist selects particular situations of a client exhibiting the observational elements of fatigue. The scientist will thus focus on observing clients for the presence of fatigue since the domain of the concept is the client. The typology thus provides an easy, clear-cut way of designating units of analysis in conceptualization. For each domain, units of analysis for concepts always exist within that domain.

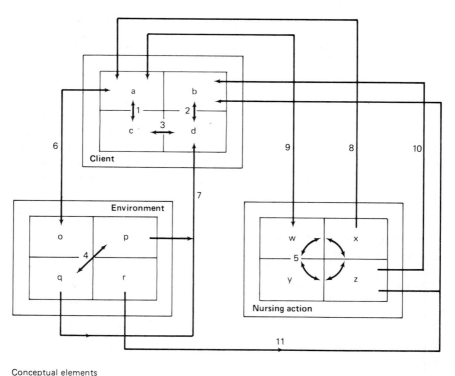

Conceptual elements

| Client | Environment | Nursing |
|---|---|---|
| a = Pain experience | o = Noise | w = Priority setting |
| b = Noncompliance | p = Family's eating habits | x = Empathic approach |
| c = Stress | q = Patient teaching conformity | y = Patient teaching |
| d = Overweight | r = Significant other | z = Negotiation |

*Figure 2.* Examples of relationships among concepts within the domains and across the domains. Numbers refer to the relationships specified in Table 4.

## UTILITY OF THE TYPOLOGY
## IN THEORETICAL DEVELOPMENT

As the second step in theoretical thinking, concepts studied and abstracted for descriptive understanding need to be exposed for their significance in theoretical formulations. The typology is useful in theoretical formulations, for the domain identification of concepts allows scientists to define the level of comprehensiveness a given theoretical formulation will have. Theoretical development in nursing is a step beyond mere conceptualization. Theoretical development involves developing sets of interlinked propositional statements for selected concepts. Since a theoretical formulation in nursing can handle concepts within or across the domains, identification of concepts with respect to the domains can show the boundaries toward which the theoretical efforts are aimed.

The typology clarifies how encompassing a theoretical formulation is in its explanatory statements. For example, a theory of cognitive dissonance in nursing is limited to explaining the phenomena in the domain of the client, whereas a theory of social support in nursing links the phenomena in the client with those in the domain of the environment. In a more global way, a general systems theory of nursing such as that proposed by Rogers encompasses in its explanatory propositions many phenomena in all three domains.

Figure 2 shows many possible theoretical clusterings of concepts among and across the domains for different types of theoretical development, albeit all theoretical linkages may be appropriate for nursing. Clusterings indicate possible propositions in theoretical systems. For example, if we designate concepts specified in the figure for each domain in the following manner, we can see many different types of theoretical formulations.

*The Domain of Client*          *The Domain of Environment*

    a = pain experience       o = noise
    b = noncompliance        p = family's eating habit
    c = stress              q = social pressure for conformity
    d = overweight         r = significant other

*The Domain of Nursing Action*

    w = priority setting
    x = empathic approach
    y = patient teaching
    z = negotiation

Thus, putting together these concepts can result in formulations of propositions. Possible relationships proposed in Table 4 serve as examples of theoretical developments linking concepts within and across the domains. These formulations implicitly show that when two or more concepts are clustered together as theoretical formulations and propositions, they tend to come together as

**TABLE 4. Examples of Theoretical Formulations Linking Concepts in Three Different Domains of Nursing**

| Domain Level | Relationship |
|---|---|
| A. Within domain | |
|   a. The domain of client | 1. Pain experience and level of stress (Theory of coping) |
| | 2. Overweight and noncompliance (Theory of balance or theory of motivation) |
| | 3. Level of stress and overweight (Theory of stress) |
|   b. The domain of environment | 4. Social pressure for conformity and significant other (Social integration theory) |
|   c. The domain of nursing action | 5. Priority assessment, empathic approach, teaching, and negotiation (Decision theory) |
| B. Across domains | |
|   a. The domains of client and environment | 6. Pain experience and noise (Theory of stress) |
| | 7. Overweight, family's eating habits, and social pressure for conformity (Reference group theory) |
|   b. The domains of client and nursing action | 8. Pain experience and empathic approach (Nursing theory of empathy) |
| | 9. Pain experience, noncompliance, overweight, and priority assessment (Nursing theory of decision) |
| | 10. Noncompliance and negotiation (Theory of contracting, theory of collaboration) |
|   c. The domains of client, environment and nursing action | 11. Noncompliance, significant other, and negotiation (Theory of influence) |

broader concepts, such as adaptation, interaction, and influence. Hence, the typology is also useful in directing the delineation of broader theoretical concepts in the process of theoretical development. These eleven examples are only some of many possible numbers of theoretical formulations linking the twelve main concepts used in this example.

As we can see in Chapter 7, not all possible linkages and clusterings of concepts are theoretically meaningful in general, nor are they specifically for nursing. Therefore, while it is not difficult to make propositional connections between concepts, it is difficult to put propositions together into a coherent system of theoretical formulations. The burden is on nursing scientists to make decisions about the nature of critical concepts and phenomena that are essential for theoretical explanations of nursing phenomena. Once essential concepts are selected, the complexity of theory evolves around the main attitudes regarding the comprehensiveness of theoretical development.

The main question for theoretical development is *to ask what needs to be explained and why such explanations might be important to nursing.* The ultimate inference in any theoretical development in nursing needs to address phenomena in the domains of client and nursing action either directly or indirectly.

## HOLISTIC AND PARTICULARISTIC MODES— CONCEPTUALIZATION WITHIN THE TYPOLOGY

For theoretical formulations in nursing, four levels of holistic conceptualization are possible and relevant, based on the three domains of the typology. These four levels of holistic theoretical systems in nursing are: (a) client; (b) environment; (c) nursing action; (d) the system of client, environment, and nursing action. In addition, within each of these four holistic levels of theoretical formulation, innumerable levels and types of a particularistic level of theoretical formulations are also possible. Table 5 lists selected concepts as "examples" of holistic and particularistic descriptions for the four levels. Scientists select and define proper levels of description for concepts chosen for specific studies within the theoretical contexts that are applied for the studies.

In many instances, the relationship between holistic and particularistic concepts for a given set of phenomena, as formulated into a proposition, takes the form of what Blalock (1969) calls "the element-class abstraction" in which a major difference in the conceptualization is in units of analysis. Such relationships and other similar relationships among different types of concepts, such as those alluded to in Figure 2, are discussed in greater detail in Chapter 7.

A word of caution is in order at this point: There is a difference between the two modes of analysis applied to *description* and the two modes of analysis applied to *explanation*. Description refers either to inductive or deductive conceptualization of phenomena for the purpose of defining the characteristics of con-

**TABLE 5. Examples of Concepts for Nursing Study According to Level of Concept Description and the Domain**

| Domain Level | Level of Concept Description | |
|---|---|---|
| | Holistic | Particularistic |
| Client | Man | Pain |
| | Health | Injury |
| | Adaptation | Anemia |
| | Coping | Depression |
| | Disability | Immobility |
| | Illness | Infection |
| | Chronicity | Edema |
| | Recidivism | Recurrent infection |
| Environment | Energy | Heat |
| | Field | Pressure |
| | Territory | Pollution |
| | Ecosystem | Noise |
| | Biosphere | Social support |
| | Milieu | Morality |
| | Time | Role-expectation |
| | | Sensory deprivation |
| | | Sensory overload |
| Nursing action | Nursing process | Communication |
| | Nursing practice | Energy exchange |
| | Interaction | Negotiation |
| | Nursing intervention | Empathy |
| | Caring | Nursing assessment |
| Client-environment-nursing action | Nursing system | Harmony |
| | Cybernetics | Attribution |
| | Transaction | Influence |

cepts. In contrast, explanation focuses on relationships between at least two phenomena or concepts. Thus, the holistic explanation aims for comprehensive understanding of changes or characteristics of the whole, while particularistic explanation is oriented toward understanding particular elements of the whole. Propositions in a holistic explanatory system tend to be global, while propositions in a particularistic explanatory system are narrower in their conceptual focus. Holistic explanations, indeed, may be aimed at grand theories. Middle range and micro-theories are aimed at particularistic explanations. This suggests that explanations within each domain are mainly particularistic explanations, whereas explanations across domains and in the system of all three domains tend to be holistic explanations.

## SUMMARY

The typology of three domains presented in this chapter and the analytic modes of holism and particularism are tools by which conceptual clarity is attained in theoretical thinking. The domain-typology aids nursing scientists in locating concepts. As presented in the following chapters, each domain poses somewhat distinct conceptual and theoretical problems and issues in nursing.

Holistic and particularistic modes of analysis as applied to the domain-typology allow theoretical thinking in nursing to be confined to certain levels of abstraction, depending upon the need for scientific explanation and investigation. If we consider nursing as inclusive of all three domains, nursing as a general concept is at the most inclusive holistic level, while each domain is in a particularistic mode. Therefore, it is a matter of scope in analysis and observation. This methodology is important for theoretical thinking. Conceptualization and related conceptual analysis require scientists to take "confined" views of the object world—the level of confinement depends upon whether one opts for a holistic mode or a particularistic one. These two frameworks are used repeatedly and consistently in analyzing concepts and examining theoretical statements throughout the book.

## BIBLIOGRAPHY

Blalock, HM, Jr. Measurement and Conceptualization Problems: The Major Obstacles to Integrating Theory and Research. *Am Sociol Rev* 44: 881–894, 1979

Blalock, HM, Jr. *Theory Construction: From Verbal to Mathematical Formulations.* Englewood Cliffs, NJ: Prentice-Hall, 1969

Carper, B. Fundamental Patterns of Knowing in Nursing. *Adv Nurs Sci* 1, No.1: 13–23, 1978

Dickoff, J, and James, P. Theory Development in Nursing. In PJ Verhonick (ed.): *Nursing Research I.* Boston: Little, Brown, 1975, pp 45–92

Donaldson, S, and Crowley, D. The Discipline of Nursing. *Nurs Outlook* 26: 113–120, 1978

Fawcett, J. The "What" of Theory Development. In *Theory Development: What, Why, How?* New York: National League of Nursing, 1978, pp 17–33

Fielo, SB. *A Summary of Integrated Nursing Theory.* New York: McGraw-Hill, 1975

Flaskerud, JH, and Halloran, EJ. Areas of Agreement in Nursing Theory Development. *Adv Nurs Sci* 3, No.1: 1–7, 1980

Glaser, B, and Strauss, A. *The Discovery of Grounded Theory*. Chicago: Aldine, 1967

Hardy, ME. Theories: Components, Development, Evaluation. *Nurs Res* 23: 100–107, 1974

Hardy, ME. Evaluating Nursing Theories. In *Theory Development: What, Why, How?* New York: National League for Nursing, 1978, pp 75–86

Jacox, A. Theory Construction in Nursing: An Overview. *Nurs Res* 23: 4–13, 1974

Murphy, JF (ed.). *Theoretical Issues in Professional Nursing*. New York: Appleton-Century-Crofts, 1971

Newman, MA. *Theory Development in Nursing*. Philadelphia: F.A. Davis, 1979

Roy, SC, and Roberts, SL. *Theory Construction in Nursing: An Adaptation Model*. Englewood Cliffs, NJ: Prentice-Hall, 1981

Schlotfeldt, R. The Need for a Conceptual Framework. In PJ Verhonick (ed.): *Nursing Research I*. Boston: Little, Brown, 1975, pp 3–24

Stevens, BJ. *Nursing Theory: Analysis, Application, Evaluation*. Boston: Little, Brown, 1979

Yura, H, and Torres, G. Today's Conceptual Frameworks Within Baccalaureate Nursing Programs. In *Faculty-Curriculum Development Part III: Conceptual Framework—Its Meaning and Function*. New York: National League for Nursing, 1975, pp 17–25

# 4

# Theoretical Analysis of Phenomena in the Domain of Client

> . . . man, you see, is to be both the knower and the object of known;
> the difficulty is that of a knower having to objectify itself and having
> then to form a just concept of what the object is.
>
> *Cassius J. Keyser*

## OVERVIEW

The primary aim of this chapter is to outline and discuss how nursing scientists might go about their search for theoretical concepts within the domain of client. The main focus is on concepts of interest to nursing that are found in this domain. This is done in three steps of discussion. Discussions in the first section attempt to clarify the essential characteristics of theoretical concepts that describe phenomena in the domain of client from the nursing perspective. The boundaries of the nursing perspective in theoretical thinking with respect to the client as the focus of attention are defined. The idea is to suggest that "the nature of the patterns and shapes one can recognize in the welter of human experience depends on one's perspective" as Blau puts it (1975, p.3).

In the second section, an attempt is made to show several different ways of abstracting the phenomena of humanity and of health in the domain of client. The concepts of humanity and health are treated here because these have been the main focal points of theoretical thinking for many nursing theorists. This section offers discussions on the approaches that are used and useful in delineating concepts based on a different intellectual scope. Approaches of delineation and abstraction are considered important in theoretical development, since it is neither necessary nor possible to observe and abstract all elements characterizing the real world in all instances. Different approaches permit abstracting selectively within proper frameworks of observation. Several nonnursing and nursing theorists' approaches in conceptualizing human person and health are brought into discussion in this section to compare and contrast the postures that emerge from different directions.

The following section provides expositions on how to analyze theoretical concepts for phenomena in the domain of client through two examples: *restlessness* and *compliance*. The purpose is to illustrate important strategies of theoretical analysis of concepts. These analyses are offered as the preludes to the development of theoretical propositions in nursing that can be used in explanations and empirical analyses. What is not dealt with in this and in the following two chapters is the advancement of specific theoretical statements of relationships among concepts in a theoretical system. The central focus in these three chapters is in abstracting, delineating, and describing phenomena of significance in theoretical terms. This step is considered a prerequisite to thinking about relationships among two or more concepts and is a necessary step for developing a theory.

## THE DOMAIN OF CLIENT IN THE NURSING PERSPECTIVE

One of the essential skills that a nurse scientist needs in order to contribute to theoretical development in nursing is the capacity to conceptualize phenomena in the client from the nursing perspective. There are almost an infinite number of concepts that describe phenomena in the client that are not significant to nursing. The nursing perspective for this domain is specifically that of "health"—health not viewed in the context of two million streptococci invading the lung tissues or of a ruptured cerebral artery, but considered in terms of *human states and behaviors of health*. Concepts and relevant phenomena in the domain of client from the nursing perspective are important to the extent that the client, the human person, is the main focus of nursing. For nursing to demonstrate its credibility and relevancy in society, it is necessary to understand, explain, and predict certain happenings in clients. These "certain happenings" and definitions of them are central to this section's theoretical thinking.

The main idea is to concentrate and direct our intellectual energy toward the study of more critical and essentially nursing-oriented concepts, selected from a vast array of possible ones. Defining a boundary is difficult because it involves a critical ability, a sense of relevance, and definite ideas about propriety for nursing. Current literature indicates that nursing scientists are approaching this boundary-definition issue in two different ways, i.e., from a holistic point of view that is global and all-encompassing, and from a particularistic point of view that is discrete and focused on selected aspects of human conditions.

The domain of client offers a vast array of human phenomena from which selections should be made for the study of appropriate and essential phenomena from the nursing perspective. As suggested in Chapter 3, the main difference between the holistic and particularistic conceptualizations of phenomena in the domain of client is in units of analysis. Holistic conceptualization in this domain necessarily has to take in the whole person as the basic unit of analysis. Particularistic conceptualization, on the other hand, takes parts or certain elements of the human person as the basic units of analysis.

Since it is somewhat arbitrary and difficult to select concepts of importance within the domain of client from the nursing perspective, I propose a scheme for categorization by which certain characteristics of human phenomena are classified for theoretical analysis in nursing. This classification scheme for the domain of client includes:

1. essentialistic concepts,
2. developmental concepts,
3. problematic concepts,
4. health-care experiential concepts.

*Essentialistic concepts* refer to those phenomena present in the client as essential characteristics and processes of human nature that are important to nursing and to human health in general. Examples of essentialistic concepts are negative feedback, homeostasis, structural integrity, and self-image.

*Developmental concepts* refer to phenomena in human development and growth. Maturation, bonding, socialization, ego-development, aging, etc., are a few examples representing developmental concepts. Both essentialistic and developmental concepts refer to normal and usual characteristics and processes that human beings experience in ordinary states of living and growing. An understanding of these phenomena will certainly aid in understanding the human person and health.

*Problematic concepts* refer to phenomena that are present in human beings as pathological or abnormal deviations from normal patternings. These concepts represent phenomena that require some type of nursing solutions. Such concepts as pain, infection, anxiety, depression, and respiratory distress are of this type. Problematic concepts have been the major focus of studies by nursing scientists, especially those who have put efforts into the development of nursing diagnosis terminologies. For this category, the term *problematic* is used *to mean problematic to nursing*. Thus, concepts such as appendicitis or bankruptcy, although these represent problematic human conditions, are not problematic concepts from the nursing perspective.

As the last group of concepts, *health-care experiential concepts* refer to phenomena that arise from people's experiences in the health-care system. This category includes such concepts as recidivism, compliance, health-belief, hospitalization, etc. This type of concept is relevant for nursing studies because it refers to selected human experiences that affect either the process of health or the contents of nursing.

Table 6 lists examples of concepts categorized according to this classification scheme and in the holistic/particularistic modes. These examples have been drawn from the current nursing literature in a casual manner, and are listed here only as typical concepts in each category according to the prototypical definitions given earlier.

**TABLE 6. Examples of Concepts in the Domain of Client for Study in the Nursing Perspective**

| Concept Type | Level of Concept Description | |
| --- | --- | --- |
| | *Holistic* | *Particularistic* |
| Essentialistic | Man<br>Health<br>Normality<br>Hope<br>Independence<br>Personality<br>Experiencing<br>Problem-<br>  solving | Coagulation<br>Respiratory compliance<br>Mutation<br>Self-image<br>Mobility<br>Dexterity<br>Ego<br>Intelligence |
| Developmental | Maturation<br>Socialization<br>Aging | Bonding<br>Ego-development<br>Moral development |
| Problematic | Stress<br>Suffering<br>Helplessness<br>Withdrawal<br>Chronicity<br>Trauma<br>Fear<br>Dysphoria<br>Fatigue<br>Anomie<br>Restlessness | Infection<br>Pain<br>Headache<br>Respiratory distress<br>Obesity<br>Amputation<br>Blindness<br>Anorexia<br>Asphyxia<br>Antisociality<br>Edema |
| Health-care experiential | Recidivism<br>Compliance<br>Institutional-<br>  ization | Nosocomial infection<br>Distrust<br>Incompatibility |

This way of classifying concepts in the domain of client focuses on client characteristics. Current development in the work for nursing diagnosis classification suggests that at present the discipline of nursing is interested more in the conceptualization of problematic and health-care experiential phenomena than in essentialistic or developmental concepts. My belief, though, is that the discipline needs to clarify conceptualization of essentialistic and developmental concepts that underpin many of the problematic and health-care experiential concepts.

This classification scheme is one way of organizing human phenomena into appropriate categories for scientific examination from the nursing perspective. Nursing is concerned with a client's behaviors, responses, and constituents to the extent that these have some bearing on his or her health, health-maintaining behaviors, and nursing requirements. While this scheme is useful for categorical thinking, and has shown that commonly studied concepts in nursing can be classified accordingly, the discipline of nursing has long been preoccupied with the ideas of the human person and of health as important conceptual issues. Major nursing theorists have struggled to present some refined ideas about these two broad concepts in their presentation of nursing theories and conceptual models. Conceptualizations of man and health are the foundations from which many other concepts in the domain of client are understood in special ways. Accordingly, conceptual notions about humans and health are usually the first and basic ideas requiring identification in the development of nursing curriculum, nursing service philosophies, and professional standards. Of all concepts relevant for inclusion within the nursing framework, the concepts of humans and health are the most essential holistic ones for theoretical thinking.

## CONCEPTUALIZATION OF MAN AND HEALTH

In a holistic posture, phenomena in the domain of client are conceptualized as systems of interlinked elements, either with respect to the nature of man or to that of health. Although there are other concepts in the holistic mode that are important to nursing, concepts of man and health stand out as the most important and essential ones for nursing. An understanding of what humans are all about and how things happen in humans is central to nursing, because the recipients of nursing actions as well as the performers of those actions are human beings. In addition, health as principally biological, that is, pertaining to life and death and states in between, is an essential property of humans. It is also the main purpose of nursing interventions.

Thus, the nursing perspective is to conceptualize a person as biopsychosocial being with an emphasis on health, and to conceptualize health as a variable state in which a person assumes certain characteristics of biological, psychological, and social functioning and feeling states. Nursing is concerned with certain types of human affairs and human well-being, i.e., health and illness. Hence, it is natural for nursing scientists to struggle for clear conceptualizations of humans and human affairs of a particular kind—health. Concepts of man and health take on proper meanings in the nursing perspective insofar as conceptualization leads to effective and scientifically valid nursing strategies.

In nursing, there has been a long history of preoccupation with a grand understanding of the human person philosophically and theoretically. One obvious reason for this preoccupation is, in a way, rooted in the profession's insistence on having philosophical stands on life, humans, health, and nursing. This value has been most clearly expressed in the accreditation criteria for nursing curriculum throughout the years. Additionally, the profession has maintained a long-standing posture that views a human being as a whole rather than as discrete details within a maze of physio-psycho-social components. Consequently, nearly all nursing theorists have supplied us with their specific visions of what a human being is and how one should understand human affairs. Likewise, we are also supplied with various conceptualizations of health by nursing theorists, motivated apparently by similar reasons.

A person is usually conceptualized in a global sense and is described in a synthesized fashion, indicating what a person is all about. Thus, nursing conceptualizations of people are generally founded on philosophical postures about human existence, and are directed toward unified views of people that are useful for nursing. This approach of aligning the conceptualization of man with the basic tenets of the profession permits development of "models of man" that are the foundations for a scientific growth of knowledge in the field. Such an approach has been used in psychology, sociology, economics, political sciences, and medicine. For example, Simon's model of man (1957) has been used in administrative science and social sciences as the basis for the fields' theoretical and empirical work. Likewise, Comte's positivistic conceptualization of a human being has influenced the early theoretical development in sociology in Europe. Models of man provide scientists with the basic attitudes and abstract tools to make detailed propositions in the development of specific theories of human beings.

In contrast to the ways models of man are developed and used in scientific fields, conceptualization of health in nursing is a movement to a somewhat particularistic level of thinking. In this sense, models of health are less global than models of man, and may develop from the main philosophical ideas of humanity but are specifically oriented to describing the nature of health, which is only one aspect of human affairs. Conceptualization of health is similar to those used for the development of conceptual models of "wealth," "knowledge," or "power," in the sense that the focus of conceptualization rests on certain characteristics of human life, not the human life itself.

These considerations point up analytical differences in the approaches for "models of man" and "models of health," although both concepts are holistic concepts for nursing. Irrespective of the approaches adopted by theorists, the focus of attention for theoretical consideration remains on those phenomena in humans related to health insofar as a model is developed from the nursing perspective. While health as a concept is implicitly inferred more often in models of man, it is explicitly defined and developed in models of health. The basic difference in these two conceptual approaches seems to be the placement of focus: The first approach for a model of man focuses on "human person," whereas the second approach for a model of health focuses specifically on "health" as the major phenomenon of interest. Thus, the two approaches pose different measurement problems in relation to health as well, in that the first approach requires measurement strategies that express the human position with respect to health, while the second approach needs to operationalize health with respect to its conceptual constituents. Regardless of the approaches adopted for explaining human phenomena in a holistic mode, models of man and health developed from the nursing perspective ultimately must be brought to bear on nursing questions. In addition, models of man and health are the basic frameworks for development of theories in nursing as well as theories in nursing on various levels and within a wide range of scope. Theoretical development for nursing thus has to be viewed to have some connections to particular models of man and health that provide the basic tenets and premises for specific delineations of theoretical statements and definitions within a theory.

These two approaches as conceptual models and theoretical systems in nursing are currently the main efforts that are being fervently pursued in nursing. It appears that the desire seems to be to develop a general nursing theory of a grand type through a model of man or a model of health. However, models of man and health are conceptual models that can be the baselines not only for theories of grand type but also for middle range and micro theories.

Although several serious attempts to develop models of humans and health are currently being made in nursing, the next section examines several other models of humans and health that have been developed by theorists in other disciplines prior to presenting the nursing models. This is done to provide a generalized baseline to compare and contrast how models of humans and health have been developed in the scientific community (including nursing), and to consider the relationships of nursing models of humans and health to other approaches. This approach of presentation is used to show that nursing models of humans and health should be examined within the broader context of the idea-systems present in the scientific community in general.

## MODELS OF MAN

It is difficult to be comprehensive in discussing models of man. Since our conceptualization of *homo sapiens* has been and will continue to be closely tied to prevailing philosophical attitudes about life, humans, and the universe, the history of dominant philosophies provides an important base for a basic understanding of how several different models of man have emerged in the recent past. For our discussion in this section, first I present only briefly several different models of man which are being debated in the scientific world and that are considered relevant to nursing. This is mainly done to provide a background for the discussion of and comparison with nursing models of man. A more comprehensive discussion follows regarding several models of man developed within the conceptual models of nursing. Philosophical and conceptual linkages between models of man developed in other relevant scientific disciplines and those developed in nursing indicate that scientific ideas in general do not arise out of a vacuum but have connections with the prevailing general paradigm of the scientific world.

Early scientific attempts at developing unified models of man can be traced back to nineteenth-century positivism. Such scientific thinkers as Huxley, Darwin, Spencer, Moleschott, and Engels influenced the culmination of a concept of humanity in which a person is mainly thought of as a species having animalistic instincts and wants. Models of man prior to the nineteenth century were so closely tied to the dominant religious beliefs and philosophies, especially backed by little biological and physical understanding of human life, that the models' influence on the conduct of human practice was profound, yet arbitrary. The arrival of positivism encouraged many scientists to try to explain human behaviors in terms of animalistic patterns. Twentieth-century logical positivism also influenced the conceptualization of humanity in many fields such as psychology, biology, and sociology. In addition, Husserl's phenomenology and various philosophical ideals of existentialism complicated theoretical thinking concerning the concepts of humanity that emerged in many directions during the twentieth century.

### Models of Man in General

As an archetype of empiricism and physicalism, the Skinnerian model of man was developed with the main focus on human behaviors. Skinnerian conceptualization is based on behaviorism that has enlarged upon the basic ideas about the need-instinct proposition of human behaviors. Both psychological and social versions of the behavioral model of man are based on the premise that human behavior is learned, maintained, extinguished, and modified by means of reward and punishment.[1] In a behavioral model, a person emits activities in a present situation based upon the experiences he or she attained either directly or vicariously as the consequences of previous activities; the consequences either reinforce or extinguish learning and repeating of activities. Behaviors are evaluated according to need/disposition or deprivation/satiation principles. Such behavioral models of man resulted from the late nineteenth and early twentieth centuries' preoccupation with a value-free, positivistic approach to the generation of scientific knowledge.

In a somewhat different orientation, Bernard, Cannon, and Selye developed a physiological conceptualization of humans. A person is viewed as striving to adapt in the most efficient manner possible to demands or stresses that are put upon the person, either as a total organism or in parts, but always striving to maintain stability within the self. Theirs was an attempt to unify a person into a whole being, opposing the scientific advances and efforts that dissected a person into organs, cells, and different functional attributes. The method of studying humans through the use of autopsy and surgical techniques in the early 1900s influenced many scientists to view humans in a dissected form. Medical and pathological atomists' conceptions of humanity have their root in such development. Although there still exist scientists whose work is based on the atomistic view of humanity, the most dominant concepts of humanity in biomedical fields are stress-adaptation models. Much of the current work in stress-adaptation models is based on the conceptual premises of the original ideas postulated by Cannon, Bernard, and Selye.[2]

René Dubos' model of man (1965) is an extension of this view of adaptation and describes all aspects of the human environment as providing ephemeral conditions. A person is thought to exercise adaptive abilities by selecting among alternatives to achieve a self-directed end, given the external conditions that are encountered at a given moment. Dubos' human, furthermore, is a product of the lasting and universal characteristics of human nature, inscribed in being, and yet is capable of establishing a personal history; thus, the person possesses both phylogenic and ontogenic adaptability. A person is seen as an organism responding to stimuli of environmental challenge in a manner that is based on rationality, i.e., that while some responses are based on the direct effects of the stimuli on the organism, most of a person's responses are usually determined not by such direct effects but by the symbolic interpretations he or she attaches to the stimuli.

Thus, Dubos' human treats and responds to actual environmental stimuli in a chained sequence of direct reactions, indirect reactions that occur as ripple effects of the direct reactions, and responses to personalized symbols that are generated by the impinging stimuli. This human trait, according to Dubos, makes the individual's responses to any environmental factors extremely personal.

Alfred Korzybski's theory of man (1921), coming from the engineering and mathematical orientation in the wake of Russell's mathematical logic and Einstein's theory of relativity, is concerned with somewhat different aspects of human nature. This model views humans as having the characteristics of time-binding power beyond the space-binding capacity of animals and the matter-energy binding property of plants. Although the language used in the description of a person in this model is highly oriented to physical sciences, it describes a person as a life form different from animals and plants, having another dimension of orientation, that of time. It is a departure from the theological and biological conceptions of humans. A person and his or her capacity are conceptualized as: (a) bound to past achievements, (b) the user of ever-increasing, inherited wisdom, and (c) the trustee of posterity. This model of man is rooted in Descartes' idea of universe in terms of space, matter, and time, and was developed with the backdrop of Einstein's proposition that links human movement in time and space to other objects in a relativistic fashion. It views humanity's basic *modus operandi* as "creative competition" by which new ideas and more goods are produced in a rational manner. By juxtaposing Korzybski's theory of man to Einstein's theory of relativity, Polakov suggested that "man measures an event from the standpoint of his own system regarded as at rest" and that a person is a relativist having a unique personal system of reference in space-time contexts (1925). An illuminating aspect of this model having a physical perspective is its conceptual likeness to Dubos' model in which personally accumulated history is stressed.

Another conceptualization of humans to emerge, rooted in Cartesian philosophy and Russell's system of mathematical logic, is economic models of man that view a person as being able to maximize preferences based on rational behaviors. The major premise of the economic model is global rationality, implying a perfect fit between a human choice and a preference, as in the game-theoretical model of vonNeuman-Morgenstern. However, Simon (1957) suggests a model that emphasizes "striving for rationality" rather than the "rationality" itself as the basis of human behavior. Simon's human strives for rationality and yet is basically oriented to a goal-satisfying rather than a goal-maximizing mode of decision-making behaviors. Simon's human makes decisions and selects choices among alternatives through a satisfying mode, a mode through which a person finds "a path that will permit satisfaction at some specified level of all of its needs" (Simon, 1957, p. 271). A satisfying mode is defined by an individual's aspirational level at the point of choice. Simon further advances his thinking on the concept of bounded rationality and its relationship to human behavior in his conceptualization of "thinking man." He recapitulates "satisficing" and "bounded rationality" as the basis of human behavior in the following way:

> ". . . a picture of Thinking Man, a creature of bounded rationality who copes with the complexity that confronts him by highly selective serial search of the environment, guided and interrupted by the demands of his motivational system, and regulated, in particular, by dynamically adjusting, multidimensional levels of aspiration."[3]

What is projected as central to human existence and human affairs in economic and administrative models of man is rationality. These models are conceptually concerned with circumscribed aspects of humans, decision-making and choice behavior. These conceptualizations are not concerned with the total organismic person as physical-biological being. For them, such biological natures are only important to the extent that they influence preferences, needs, and evaluations of utilities. Therefore, human aspects other than rationality are only contextual to studying the processes through which a person handles himself and the external factors. If we were to apply these models of man directly to viewing the client in the nursing perspective, the theoretical explanations of human phenomena will be limited to choice-behaviors. Thus, such a model is useful only in studying particularistic phenomena in the domain of client.

In addition to the behavioral model discussed earlier, there are several different concepts of the psychological model of man. Three views stand out distinctively, indicating different orientations. The psychoanalytic models of man advanced by Freud and reformulated by many scientists[4] are based on the idea of organizational and dominational relationships among different psychological elements in humanity. The id (or the instinct), the ego (the consciousness), and the superego are the main human elements that determine self-generated actions and a person's relations to the world outside. Ego as consciousness plays an important role in attaining, maintaining, and controlling human responses in the psychoanalytic models of man. A person's actions are the extensions of suppressions of the id's wants and the superego's controls by the consciousness, and yet expressed by the dominations obtained by different aspects of the personality for pleasure and power.

On the other hand, Maslow (1967 and 1973) attempts to generate an idea of humanity by interfacing human needs that are basically psychological in nature with the biological makeup of the human organism. Maslow's concept of a person as an organism that is oriented to self-regulation, self-government, and self-choice is akin to the rationalist view of humanity. However, it is based on the notion that human needs are fundamentally biological. He classifies human needs into two types: (a) the basic needs including safety and protection, belongingness, love, respect, self-esteem, identity, and self-actualization; and (b) the meta-needs including truth, goodness, beauty, justice, order, law, unity, etc. These needs are seen tied to the structure of the human organism itself. He conceptualizes variations in human conditions according to satisfaction and deprivation of need, and views deprivation as the cause for disease or illness.

Gestalt psychologists' view of a person as a personalistic, holistic being is a more recent concept of humanity in psychology. This concept of unitary human being suggests that human activities are produced by integrated efforts of a person to express what he or she knows and how he or she deals with this knowledge within the context of given biological conditions. The Gestalt person is understood not in his or her componental characteristics but as the whole depicted in his or her experience and behaviors.

Psychological models of man also have limiting explanatory use for human phenomena in the nursing perspective. Only selected phenomena in the client can be studied within theoretical systems that are based on psychological models of man for nursing.

Of course, there are many more models of man that have been proposed by scientists in different disciplinary orientations. For example, Parsons' model of social humanity is composed of personality and organism, acting and interacting with objects and other human beings in the social world. A person acts and interacts within given cognitive, cathectic, and evaluative motivations. The Parsonian individual is a product of integration of cultural values and social norms. Furthermore, human deviant behaviors are viewed in the context of functionality to the social systems rather than to the individual's motivations or needs. A social person thus is a constrained being, acting within the limits of individual, social, and cultural standards and expectations.

Another example is a biomedical model. In addition to the dissected view of human system as a biological being, there has been a growing interest in medical fields for a development of conceptualization of humanity that encompasses bioethical issues that have raised many moral questions in the practice of health care in recent years. In an attempt to view humanity in the context of biomedical ethics, Fletcher (1979) proposes a composite human model. He specifies the necessary characteristics of a human person in terms of: (a) minimum intelligence, (b) self-awareness, (c) self-control, (d) a sense of time, (e) a sense of futurity, (f) a sense of the past, (g) the capacity to relate to others, (h) concern for others, (i) communicability, (j) control of existence and freedom, (k) curiosity, (l) change and changeability, (m) balance of rationality and feeling, (n) idiosyncracy and individuality, (o) neocortical function, (p) not non- or antiartificial, (q) not essentially parental, (r) not essentially sexual, (s) not a bundle of rights, and (t) not a worshipper. This model raises several moral and ethical questions regarding the values of life and existence. Although such a model can create a great deal of controversy and discussion, it can serve scientists to view human life and human existence from quite different perspectives. More importantly, when such a model is applied to human services, there are many practice implications. In any event, such a model at least provides a framework upon which evaluation of human nature may begin and questions related to human interventions are addressed.

These are but some of the eclectic examples of models of man in a variety of scientific fields that suggest varied viewpoints and different angles of vision. As this cursory review of such models suggests, our conceptions of humanity are closely related to philosophical ideas about meanings attached to differentiating the subjective from the objective and about a person's relations to the world and herself or himself. Scientific advancement and technology, as well as the dominant modes of scientific investigation, also influence our ideas about human nature, capacities, and variabilities. Disclosures briefly discussed in these pages indicate that a person may appear differently when objectified with the tinted glasses of biologist, psychologist, sociologist, mathematician, or physician. Yet a person may also be perceived in the same manner even among scientists of different disciplinary orientations and of varying perspectives. It is also obvious that scientists use their conceptual models of man for different purposes, i.e., for development of a theory of man, an ethical basis of scientific inquiry, a framework for human intervention, or as a starting point for philosophical discourse.

These examples also indicate that models of man conceptualized in other disciplines have limited theoretical utility for nursing if they are applied directly to nursing without expansion or modification. This enlightens our thinking and directs us toward developing nursing models of man. For nursing explanations, it is necessary to have nursing models of man, the contributions to the discipline of nursing of theoretical developments in other fields for models of man notwithstanding. The specific nature of essential phenomena in nursing within the domain of client requires conceptualization of humanity that addresses such specific nature.

### Nursing Models of Man

In nursing, then, what should a model of man describe? Nursing models of man tend to describe humanity with respect to placement in and operations related to health and well-being. Conceptual models proposed by Rogers, Roy, and Johnson have attempted to do this. I shall attempt at this point to summarize the mental images that these nursing theorists have projected in their models of man. Of course, it needs to be made clear that these theorists describe their ideas in an implicit manner and do not call their conceptualizations of humanity, models. Health is usually the major theme handled in nursing models of man as the essential descriptive characteristics of humanity. The current conceptualization of humanity in nursing models can be categorized into four major types according to their views of health as an essential human condition: (a) person attaining health through "balance," (b) human "process" as the basis of health, (c) human "configuration" as the basis of health, and (d) human health expressed as "aggregation" of parts.

This idea of differentiating conceptual approaches to formulating models of man in terms of *balance, process, configuration,* and *aggregation* is proposed here in order to attain a clear mental picture of human phenomena. By introducing this classification, we are also able to compare nursing human models with those discussed earlier. Balance model is a conceptualization in which human phenomena are considered in terms of integration and stability. Selye's stress model of man is a balance model in which human phenomena are mainly considered with respect to equilibrium.

Process model is a conceptualization in which human phenomena are explained as everchanging, continuing activities. Dubos' adaptive model of man is of this kind in which a person is depicted as an everadapting, growing entity. The configuration model refers to a conceptualization of human phenomena in which integration among different elements and subsystems is taken to be the major characteristic. Gestalt human models are of this type.

The aggregation model is a conceptualization in which a person is viewed as an entity of different elements. Human phenomena are expressed as the additiveness of different elements that make up a person. Biological and medical models of man tend to take this form of conceptualization of humanity.

Johnson's behavioral system is an example of the balance model. Johnson (1980) refers to humanity as a behavioral system comprised of patterned, repetitive, and purposeful ways of behaving. Human behaviors are formed into an organized and integrated functional unit. Human health is implicitly expressed as the state of behavioral system balance and dynamic stability. According to Johnson, it is not the nature of properties or state of a person that is central to his or her health and existence, but it is the system of behaviors as parts of an organized and integrated whole that is. Thus, although labeled as a behavioral model, its premises are quite variant from the classical behavioral models of reinforcement and extinction. This concept of balance as the expression of health is akin to the systems theorists' view of humanity that considers a person as striving to attain the maximum balance and homeostasis. From the latter's perspective, a system's adaptiveness with respect to stability is the central process for an explanation of variants in system-states, whether expressed in terms of behaviors or states.

Although Johnson identifies subsystems within the human behavioral system, it is ultimately the behavior as a whole that is the phenomenon of interest to her. Johnson states that this conceptualization is not intended to provide a framework for marking the boundary of what aspects of the behavioral system are appropriate for the perspective of nursing. An implicit inference in the model is that any possible or actual imbalance or deviation from the dynamic stability of the behavioral system is a potential target for nursing intervention. However, the specific types of behaviors or imbalances as the main targets for nursing intervention are neither clearly indicated nor implicitly stated.

The conceptual ideas projected in Rogers' model of unitary man are related to process. Rogers (1970 and 1980) conceptualizes a person as continually renewing his or her patterns of life toward increasing complexity and negentropy. The patterns of life process are seen as manifested through a person's mutual, simultaneous interactions with the environment in the forms of helicy, resonancy, and complementarity.[5] Rogers' human, having an everexpanding and contracting human field, is in the process of interchange with the environmental field in a reciprocal fashion; such interchange is based on the homeodynamic principles of complementarity, helicy, and resonancy. In his or her personal evolution in a given space and through time, a person adopts these forms of interactive exchange of energy. These are basic forms of life processes for an increased organization and patterning in one's field-relations and interchanges with the environmental field.

Rogers depicts a person as not having specific goals in his or her evolutionary journey through life, except for the increasing complexity in organization and patterning, as the law of human developmental process. Furthermore, a person's goals in the life-process are probabilistic rather than deterministic. This means that a person's goals in life process change with the progression of the process itself, and that goals are revised and formulated according to changes in personal evolution. What is most explicit in this model is the unity of a person as interacting-being, having personal identity and existence defined by his or her relationships with the environment. Thus, it is not possible to understand Rogers' human evolutionary identity or process without having the knowledge of the characteristics of the environmental field or the person's relationships with it. Rogers also identifies seven qualities: wholeness, openness, unidirectionality, pattern, organization, sentience, and thought as the basic properties of the life processes that determine the ways complementarity, helicy, and resonancy in interchange are adopted in given situations. Thus, Rogers' human is an everchanging entity whose characteristics are not determined by genetic givens, destiny, or predetermined patterns of growth, but are influenced in dynamic ways by the changing nature of his or her environment, the changing nature of self, and the evolving nature of interchange between them. Goals of life are never fixed, nor are the patterns of change that are possible for an individual's life.

Rogers implies that health is expressed as the process of life in its totality. She postulates that nursing seeks to (a) strengthen the human-environment symmetry, (b) promote synchronic interaction between a person and his or her environment, (c) strengthen the coherence and integrity of the human field, and (d) direct repatterning of the human and environmental fields for more effective fulfillment of life's capabilities and realization of maximum health potential (1970). The patterns of life process that an individual attains express whether or not he or she has realized his or her health potential. What is not specified in the model is an explicit definition of "health potential." Rogers' implicit notion of health stands for a person in a state of continuing, maturational complexities, not defined by any standardized expectations, but expressed only as evolutionary, sequential happenings. To Rogers, the human-environment field is an entity that generates organization and patterning; it is treated as though it has a consciousness or goal-directedness for an everincreasing organization and patterning. The model gives the impression that the human-environment integrity is as critical for human existence as a person's integrity itself.

In the Roy Adaptation Model (1970, 1976, and 1981), a person is perceived as an adaptive system receiving inputs identified as stimuli from the external environment and as generated by the self, processing them by internal and feedback processes inherent in an individual's everchanging abilities, and producing outputs as either adaptive or ineffective responses.[6] To Roy, adaptation has a positive connotation, a state of "all systems go," a "green light" in specific relation to what is happening to the person at a given moment. Roy's human responds to stimuli in four basic adaptive modes: (a) physiological needs, (b) self-concept, (c) role-function, and (d) interdependence. Adaptive or ineffective responses result from the functioning of two basic mechanisms of controlling and responding: regulator and cognator.

Because Roy conceptualizes a person as having four distinct modes for adapting to stimuli, the concept of humanity according to this model is that of configuration, although there is an element of balance suggested in the model. A person is depicted as a configuration of responses in four adaptive modes. Thus, human responses are the major phenomena of interest in Roy's model and are analyzed in terms of their adaptiveness in relation to four modes in an individual. Health, then, is relative to the person's responses to stimuli that promote the person's general goals of survival, growth, reproduction, and mastery, manifested within each adaptive mode. A person who responds ineffectively to stimuli is seen as capturing and spending energy for the particular set of stimuli, exhibiting behaviors that are incongruent with the valued goals. Roy's human is a reactive entity whose basic mechanisms become activitated in response to impinging stimuli. The characteristics of creativity and self-determination are not emphasized in the model.

These three nursing models of man are contrasted here in order to provide concepts of humanity that are quite different from one another yet have significant identification in the nursing perspective. These nursing theorists' ideas suggest that in the nursing perspective a person may be described in terms of the nature of his or her behaviors ( Johnson), the level of complexity in organization and patterns exhibited in the person's relations with the environment (Rogers), or the characteristics of responses to stimuli impinging on the person depicted either as adaptive or ineffective (Roy). As shown here, the concepts of balance, process, configuration, and aggregation as the distinguishing characteristics of human models can only be used to identify the dominant features of models rather than to label them as confined to specific types.

As indicated in these discussions, it is possible, then, to imagine a room with nursing scientists perceiving the client in many different ways, and analyzing health problems with different conceptual orientations. Rogers will wonder about the size, shape, and quality of the client's energy field and how the nurse's presence as an element in the environmental field affects the client's interchanges with the external world. Johnson's posture will be that of analyzing the client's behaviors in terms of the integration as a whole person-system. In contrast, Roy will evaluate the client's responses to the situation as adaptive or ineffective and identify the focal, contextual, and residual stimuli that cause deficits in the adaptive responses.

As Barrett (1978) suggested, a person becomes *Janus,* and each scientist or theorist or philosopher is imprisoned in his or her seat for a view of particular features. The question is whether a scientist should get up from his or her seat and walk around to obtain views of all the features from different angles, or should remain in one position in order to attain an indepth understanding of that one particular feature. It is certainly a paradox for scientists who wish to be comprehensive in the understanding of a phenomenon and at the same time desire to gain a detailed knowledge of a single aspect of that phenomenon.

The crux of the matter is in the complexities: A person eats, plays, and fights; laughs and cries; does good for others and commits sins; falls in love and falls out of love; makes friends and seeks solitude; is happy, sad, and plainly content; makes decisions and follows the decisions of others blindly; and is healthy, ill, disabled, and dying. All these and more make the conceptualization of a person difficult. Nursing models of man, therefore, can at least confine our theoretical interests to selected human features.

## MODELS OF HEALTH

Another holistic approach to conceptualizing phenomena in the domain of client has been specified earlier as models of health. The theoretical focus of this approach in nursing is to view health as having particular meanings for nursing actions. Thus, in this approach, *health* would be defined in terms of nursing care needs and nursing interventions. Although health as a concept is rather global, compared to the concept of a person, it encompasses rather selected sorts of phenomena in humans. Because of this, many models of man contain basic notions about the phenomena of health, as indicated in the discussions presented in the preceding section. Health represents a circumscribed aspect of human phenomena and can be conceptualized in more particularistic modes. The literature indicates that models of health may be differentiated into two distinct types: structural models and functional models.

Structural models of health are oriented to looking at human structures and properties as the major indicators of the phenomena of health. In contrast, functional models of health view health as intrinsically tied to human functioning. In this section, models are examined according to these two types. Models of health proposed by scientists of other disciplines as well as by nursing theorists are examined together in this section according to the types to which the models are classified.

### Structural Models of Health
The structural, property-oriented approaches are rooted in the long history of considering "health" as opposite to sickness, disease, and illness, beginning with the ancient ideas (i.e., Egyptian and Greek) about the relationships between the way one feels and the nature of bodily constituents. Structural models of health are oriented to distinguishing the "normal" nature and constitution of elements in a human person, especially in the body—the physical being—and the deviations that exist that influence the way a person feels, per-

forms duties, and behaves. In general, these models are clinically and/or medically oriented models, in which causes for changes and deviations are the main epistemological interests.

Thus, for the conceptualization of health in such approaches, it is essential to know what causes deviations, hence the development of a string of theories of pathophysiological explanations, starting with early demonic theories of disease. Historically, many of the medically oriented theories of disease belong to this type of approach: Examples are Galen's theory of humoral balance as the basis of diseased states; the miasmic theory of illness of eighteenth century by which the production of disease is attributed to invasion of the body by earthly, noxious miasma; the germ theory of nineteenth and early twentieth centuries; general adaptation syndrome as the basis of stress/adaptation; and the current biochemical theories of pathology.

Health in a structural model is indicated by signs and symptoms a person experiences or exhibits. These are considered changes and deviations in the human elements and structures. Currently, there are two general structural models of health: clinical model and adaptation model.

*Clinical models,* generally having a historical linkage to earlier conceptualizations of "disease" in medicine, are oriented to explaining health in pathological terms. Clinical models view health as a state in which there is an absence of abnormal signs and symptoms and as an opposite state of "diseased." In a diseased state, a person is in acquisition of an undesirable, abnormal, or deviant entity or property in human structures with specific known or unknown etiologies.

The terms *signs* and *symptoms* in this context have negative, undesirable connotations. While current clinical models in general have reconciled with the unified view of a human as a free-flowing integration of mind and body, there is a tendency in clinical models to have a deterministic view of what might go wrong with human nature in given situations. The earlier conceptualizations of health in clinical models were implicitly based on the dualism of the "psyche" (the mind) and the "soma" (the body). Incorporation of the ideas on psychosomatic interdependence is a more recent development in clinical models. Yet the recent interest in psychopharmacological research indicates persisting adherence of clinical models to physicalism as the major philosophical orientation.

The deterministic view in clinical models is evident in the continuing search for causal factors for diseases. Clinical models usually assume the scientific posture that seeks to identify and understand characteristics of diseased states as primary for correcting the diseased states.

*Adaptation models* are of more recent development. The concept of general adaptation syndrome (Selye, 1956 and 1976) popularized the view of health in relation to an individual's responses and behaviors to stresses and noxious stimuli. Health in these models is conceptualized as a state of coping and adapting within a continuously changing environment. Health indicates that a person maintains his or her integrity of structures and yet changes his or her nature and behaviors to respond effectively to situational demands. Engel (1970) suggests that health and disease are phases that result as the human organism strives to master and handle stresses that are continually posed by environments on multiple levels, i.e., cellular, chemical, physiological, and behavioral levels. He views a state of health as when an organism functions effectively as a whole, fulfilling needs, successfully responding to the requirements of the environment, and pursuing its biological destiny, including growth and reproduction (Engel, 1975). This state of health is specifically tied to the adaptation that occurs in the human organism.

Adolf Myer's work on stressful life events, the framework of Howard and Scott (1965), and the work of Hinkle (1961) and Wolff (1962) propose ecologically oriented adaptation models of health in which health is viewed as adjustments to one's social environment and occurrences in life situations. Such ecologically oriented adaptation models consider the ecological influences as structurally demanding and causing changes in the structures of adaptation.

Fabrega (1974) proposes a somewhat different adaptation model, which he calls a "phenomenologic" view of health and disease. The basic assumption is that disease needs to be understood in the context of an individual's subjective experiences. Such subjective experiences are thought to be shaped by social and cultural patterns. Characteristics of disease in the phenomenologic model encompass changes in the state of being, such as in the state of feeling, thought, self-definition, impulses, etc. These changes are seen as discontinuous with everyday affairs and are believed to be caused by socioculturally defined agents and circumstances. The main "change" of structure of interest to Fabrega is an altered concept of self-identity. In a phenomenologic sense, an altered self-identity is defined as disturbed feelings, bodily sensations, beliefs about how the body functions, self-derogatory convictions, imputations of moral guilt, etc. As the major form of disease state, it is inclusive of discomfort, disability, discreditation, and danger according to Fabrega (1974).

Among nursing models in which health is considered as a concept, Roy's adaptation model treats health as a state of structural characteristics in adaptive processes (1981). Roy suggests that a state of health is possible for a person who is adaptive. A person is healthy when he or she is able to direct energies to respond to multiple stimuli of life rather than expanding and concentrating on one set of stimuli. In essence, Roy's model views health as having certain property and structural characteristics in an individual organism. A state of health is attained when an individual receives an appropriate type and amount of stimuli and has structural integrity in adaptive modes and mechanisms.

Health in structural models is operationalized and measured most appropriately in terms of feeling-states, perceptions, and sign/symptom complexes. State-characteristics that are considered the indicators of health in these models are: (a) measured objectively and compared to the established norms as the expression of "healthy" state, as in the clinical measurements of blood pressure, body weight, level of hemoglobin, size of liver; (b) expressed as experiences and perceptions, as in feelings of pain, headache, depression, fatigue, discomfort, respiratory distress; or (c) assessed as behaviors of adaptation, as in adaptive versus maladaptive behaviors, negative versus positive responses, enhancing versus destroying behaviors.

Instruments developed currently with this approach in the conceptualization of health are found in the works by Given, Simoni, and Gallin (1977); Kennedy, Northcott, and Kinzel (1978); and Wan (1976), among many others. In the same tradition, Turnbull (1976) treats health for nursing in a strictly structural perspective. A measurement of wellness and health is expressed in terms of intactness, symmetry, nourishment, and productivity. Structural models of health are thus oriented to describing health in terms of changes that are present in human structures producing variations in feeling states, behaviors, and appearances of the structures.

## Functional Models of Health

Functional models begin with a premise that health is a state of variability in human functioning. The functionalists' approaches view dimensions of health and variations in the state of health in terms of a human ability to perform required functions. Optimum health refers to the normative reference point of desired capacity and functioning.

Naegel (1970) perceives health as "a condition necessary for the realization of two of our regnant values: mastery of the world and fun." Health as a state allows one to do what one wants to do and to be what one wants to be. As an opposite state, illness is seen to impede activity and to limit one's autonomy, and it is a state of frustration and deprivation. In addition, Naegel sees health as a moral good that is desired by all but vaguely defined: health is part of the condition of participation in social life as a valued state. In this view, health is globally described in social, functional terms. Health is a state in which a person is able to participate in the affairs of the world and the affairs of self with the freedom of the individual. To Naegel, autonomy is the basic functional requirement for an individual's freedom of pursuit, and health is the end-state in which the individual's autonomy can be enjoyed.

If we are to designate Naegel's concept of health as a functionalist's orientation in an individualistic sense, then Parsons' concept of health is a functionalist's approach in a social sense. Parsons (1950 and 1958) conceptualizes health as a socially desirable and normative state that is functionally important to the social system. To Parsons, health is a functional requirement for maintaining integration in the social system in an aggregated form. From this assumption, an individual's health is defined in terms of his or her capacities to assume roles and perform essential social tasks satisfactorily. Twaddle (1974) consolidates both the biological and sociological meanings of functioning into a more inclusive conceptualization of health. In addition, health is a state labeled by self and others according to Twaddle.

Twaddle proposes the following postulates as the essential ideas about health and illness:

1. Health and illness are defined normatively and refer to "standards of adequacy relative to capacities, feeling states, and biological functioning needed for the performance of those activities expected of members of a society," and yet deviations from the norms are rather ambiguously defined by the society.
2. Health and illness are designated according to the norms of functioning in the biological context, in that parameters of biological functioning are used as the criteria designating the health status.
3. The norms for differential labeling and designation of health status are not consistently applied to social groups, in that the norms tend to be differentially interpreted among different social groups, social situations, and times, and differently applied by different individuals.[7]

Correspondingly, health is a designated state in which adequacy in one's capacities for role and task performance is judged by self and others against normative and socially held standards. What is most essential for these functional approaches, then, is the definition of "normal" or "expected" human functioning and capacity for functioning. Insofar as a person is capable of functioning as expected and adequately, an enlarged heart, an absence of a kidney, or the presence of discomfort and pain is not essential to this conceptualization of health. Engelhardt (1976) also notes that the conceptions of health and illness are tied to our ideologies and expectations concerning the world, in that we identify and judge certain states as illnesses according to what we consider as dysfunctional, deformed, or violating the norms of a reasonable expectation with regard to freedom of action on our part as humans. He considers it an instance of "hubris." Many recent studies indicating different evaluative standards of health applied to the general adult population and those applied to the aged suggest that differential criteria for evaluation of health status do exist for subpopulation categories.

The functional approaches have been used quite frequently in health services research. Efforts to develop indicators of health that depart from the classical, clinical measurements of abnormalities have evolved into several indices of health that are based on functioning. For example, as a most comprehensive approach, the Rand Health Insurance Study (1979) has used physical, social, and psychological functioning as the basis for the development of health status indicators. Kaplan, Bush, and Berry (1976) also carried out a survey study in which normative designations of functioning capacities were assessed in order to use them as a reference guide for health-status designations. The long-standing use of activities of daily living scales in rehabilitation and gerontology is an example of application of the functional approaches for health assessment.

In nursing, Orem's self-care model is a version of a functional model of health. Orem conceptualizes health in relation to self-care deficits, which are expressed as deficiencies in any one of the self-care foci identified in three categories of universal, developmental, and health-deviation self-care types (1980). Orem views health as the following:

> Health includes that which makes a person human (form of mental life), operating in conjunction with physiological and psychophysiological mechanisms, and a material structure (a biologic life), and in relation to and interaction with other human beings (interpersonal and social life).[8]

Health is a state of wholeness or integrity of the person in terms of his or her capacity to provide self-care. Since Orem views a human being as a unity functioning biologically, symbolically, and socially, one has to be able to perform deliberate actions to be functional and healthy. Health is thus attained by sufficient and satisfactory self-care actions responding to varying demands for attention to self. Effectively performed self-care action contributes to human integrity, human functioning, and human development. Orem further proposes that the client's health in the nursing perspective should be considered according to three types of self-care requisites (1980). Universal self-care requisites are considered to have six foci: (a) air, water, and food; (b) excrement; (c) activity and rest; (d) solitude and interaction; (e) hazards to life and well-being; and (f) normalcy. Developmental self-care requisites encompass two categories: (a) conditions that support life processes and promote the process of development; and (b) provisions for preventing exposure to deleterious conditions or for developing strategies to deal with harmful conditions. Health-care deviation self-care requisites are related to six categories: (a) preventive and proactive health-seeking; (b) therapeutic; (c) compliant to medical measures; (d) awareness of adverse effects of health-care; (e) self-concept generating; and (f) accepting and adjusting to health deviation consequences. Thus, self-care is the functional capacity to handle such requirements and is considered as deliberate action, either routine or programmed. Usually, self-care actions performed in daily living become routine, while new self-care actions have to be learned in response to given, specific demands.

Although Orem's attempt is to conceptualize health in a nursing frame of reference, moving away from medical, psychological, and sociological orientations, the self-care model suffers from its implicit assumptions of "unbounded rationality" as the basis for choice of actions and of "deliberateness" in choices as well as in actions. What is not handled adequately in the conceptualization of the model is the role of unconscious, reflexive, and autonomic human responses that define a person's functional capacities that are responsible for many types of self-care activities.

As shown in these discussions of various models of health, a purely structural or functional conceptualization of health appears to be inadequate and incomplete in abstracting the complex phenomena of health. Recent interests in applying the general systems approaches to conceptualization of health are attempts to overcome such inadequacies.

Departing from the conventional perspectives and approaches presented in the preceding section, Newman (1979) proposes a theory of health, based on Rogers' model of unitary man. Newman's basic assumptions regarding health, which is viewed as the synthesis of disease at one end and nondisease on the other, are six-fold:

1. Health encompasses conditions of illness or pathology that are accompanied by varying degrees of incapacitation.
2. Conditions of illness or pathology are manifestations of the total pattern of the individual.
3. The manifested patterns of the individual precede structural or functional changes.
4. The manifested patterns of the individual are not pathology itself, and thus removal of pathology in itself will not change the patterns of the individual.
5. Being ill is healthful when it is the only way an individual's patterns can manifest in a given life process situation.
6. Health is the expansion of consciousness and is the totality of the life process.[9]

To Newman, the phenomena of health constitute the concepts of movement, time, space, and consciousness. Newman poses five general propositions, considering the expansion of consciousness as the expression of health. Hence, the processes that specify how an individual expands consciousness will explain how an individual progresses in life with respect to health.

Newman considers time and space as the basis of life processes, having a complementary relationship. Time and space are postulated to be in a complementary elasticity by which an individual moves about in relation to space and time. This suggests that an individual compensates for a loss in space with a gain in time and vice versa. Therefore, the patterns of an individual are manifested through this complementary process. Yet space and time as objective world elements are meaningless to an individual until one's position in it is expressed by movement.

To Newman, the personal reality comes into existence via patterns of movement. The meanings of space and time are relative to movements of self and perceived others. In addition, the patterns of movement are expressed within the conscious recognition of body and self. Thus, expressions of self are manifested in movements, and time is "possessed" by an individual through the patterns of movement one develops. Furthermore, since consciousness means awareness of the life context in space-time dimensions, time measures the level of expanded consciousness.

This conceptualization departs in several ways from the conventional views of health in nursing. To begin with, health is neither viewed in relation to structural integrity nor to functional competency. It is not a property concept, but a process concept. Health is an expression of the level to which an individual's consciousness has expanded and is expanding, influencing the awareness of self, which in turn determines the ways the individual moves within subjective time and space. Time and space are media within which an individual expands self through movement and consciousness. Thus, health is a process in which one finds individualized yet evolving patterns of movement and consciousness, defining and claiming "possessed" and "private" space and time from those that are present in the object world. Indeed, this conceptualization is revolutionary and requires a set of different world views. In this view, health is holistic, transcending the notions of illness, disease, or even body and mind. It nearly means life itself; therefore, the conceptualization suffers from a lack of specificity. If health is the processes of life, it is conceived interchangeably with the concept of life. According to this conceptualization of health, a state of health cannot be differentiated from a state of life. In addition, this concept equates health with a state of consciousness, yet the meaning of consciousness is not explicitly defined in the theory. If consciousness is "knowing," this conceptualization also disregards that aspect of human life controlled, regulated, and promoted by the reflexive, autonomic, and unconscious responses. Consciousness equated with the concept of life also raises a philosophical question regarding the intrinsic value of human existence. Certainly, Newman's theory of health opens the way for many other possible revolutionary conceptualizations of health that may be more particularly fitting to theoretical thinking in nursing.

However, these discussions indicate that what is most critical in studying the phenomena of health rests not on the development of a unified concept of health, but on the understanding that different approaches of conceptualization of health, e.g., structuralism, functionalism, general systems approach, essentialism, or relativism, will lead to different sets of theoretical ideas and explanations. Accordingly, health may be understood and explained in relation to such concepts as attitude, value, quality of life, experience, stressful life events, attribution, help-seeking behavior, energy expansion, sensory deprivation, self-image, etc.

This section has presented diverse conceptual thinking about humanity and health. As indicated earlier, the nursing perspective needs to steer our conceptual development and theoretical analysis to those areas of human affairs and human nature related to health. For nursing to make theoretical sense as a field, it is necessary to develop conceptual and theoretical approaches that can be used for nursing's understanding of human health. At the same time, truly fruitful theoretical advancements may not result directly from such holistic conceptualizations of humanity and health, but from more focused approaches that are developed to understand more particularistic aspects of humanity and health. This idea is in line with the assertion that nursing may benefit more at the present time by developing middle range theories of nursing rather than by trying to muddle through grand conceptualizations of humanity and health. What is needed in developing middle range theories of nursing is a fundamental philosophy about human life and health rather than a well-developed conceptual model.

## SELECTED CONCEPTUAL ANALYSIS:
## RESTLESSNESS AND COMPLIANCE

In the first section of this chapter, a list of concepts in the domain of client as examples for the nursing perspective was presented. In this section, conceptual analysis of two selected concepts in the domain of client are presented. The main purpose of this section is to show how a first-level analytical approach is used to gain conceptual and empirical understanding of phenomena. Two concepts, *restlessness* and *compliance,* are treated as examples for clarifying conceptual ideas about them and their relevance in the framework of nursing. Restlessness is selected as an example of a ''problematic'' concept, and compliance is selected as an example of a ''health-care experiential'' concept. Each concept is analyzed with respect to (a) definitional clarification and conceptual meanings as reflected in the literature, (b) measurement and operationalization of concepts as a step toward an empirical analysis, and (c) the concept's relationships with other concepts that are important in nursing. The strategy and rationale for the conceptual analysis were discussed in detail in Chapter 2, and that rationale is adopted in this section for the analyses of restlessness and compliance. The specific reasons for selecting these two concepts are meaningless for actual presentations and have no significance to our exercises in theoretical thinking. However, there is a contrast in the level and richness of conceptual development for these two concepts: Restlessness as a concept has received very little scientific attention, while compliance has been studied not only by nursing scientists but also scientists in other behavioral and social sciences during the past decade.

## RESTLESSNESS

*Scenario*
Ellen Austin, R.N., who is a team leader for this unit of ten semicritically ill patients reports about the experiences during the night of two patients: Mrs. Jane Turcotte is a 32-year-old woman who was admitted to the hospital with

abdominal and chest injuries resulting from an automobile accident six days ago; Mr. Thomas Taylor is a 68-year-old patient who is diabetic and has chronic obstructive lung disease, and has been on this unit for the past ten days. Ms. Austin reports:

"Mrs. Turcotte had a very restless night. I do not think she slept even ten minutes. She thrashed about the bed all night long, was agitated and restless. She received the pain medication and the sedative, but these didn't induce her to rest. She took off her TEDS several times, almost pulled off her dressing, and attempted to get out of the bed. I stayed with her for a while, which seemed to calm her down a little. Mr. Taylor was out of his bed and walked up and down the corridor more than ten times during the night. He would get into the bed, then get up and sit in the chair, and then walk. This was repeated many times. He took a dose of sleeping medication early in the evening and did not want it repeated. He must be exhausted this morning. I asked him why he was so restless. He couldn't tell me the reason."

## Definition

*Restlessness* is most commonly used in the adjective form to describe people's behaviors of agitation. Although the phenomenon of restlessness seems to be a frequent occurrence, it has not been studied extensively as a distinct concept in the literature. Yet the phenomenon of restlessness is found in ordinary life situations and in patients' experiences. We have seen many patients in hospitals, nursing homes, and clinics in a state of restlessness and agitation. We also have experienced restless moments and hours ourselves when we found ourselves wandering about the house without aim, and with a feeling of uneasiness and agitation. Norris (1975) found in her literature review that restless behaviors are found in animals in preparation for migration or hybernation. As described in the above scenario, there are many forms of behaviors that are associated with restlessness.

*Agitation* is the most commonly used term in combination with restlessness to describe a behavioral state that includes aimless, roving, or wandering movements of the body or extremities. English and English (1958) define restlessness as "a tendency to aimless and constantly changing movements," and define agitation as "a condition of tense and irrepressible activity, usually rather 'fussy' and anxious." Barnes (1979) defines agitation as "a broad behavioral term connoting excessive motor activity, often nonpurposeful in nature, and commonly associated with feelings of internal tension, irritability, hostility and belligerency." A person in a state of restlessness tends to move about without purpose, with an unspecified feeling of uneasiness and tension. It is a behavioral state of motor activity accompanied with specific kinds of emotional experiences, and thus is a property concept. Norris (1975) suggests that restlessness may be specified by behavioral indicators: (a) increased, repetitive, aimless skeletomuscular activities; (b) urgency in repeating the activities; and (c) increased muscle tones of body, face, or both. These definitions suggest that restlessness is a state of behavioral movements of muscles, combined with an uneasy feeling state.

Restlessness is a "problematic" concept because it represents a state that requires our questioning of its causes, and because it is an undesirable, troublesome state requiring some form of solution, especially when it lasts for a long duration. Although restlessness of a short duration, the passing restlessness we experience in everyday life, is one in the normal repertoire of human behavioral experiences, when it exists in a person for a prolonged duration or is exaggerated in its intensity as apparent in the two patients in the scenario, the phenomenon acquires a pathologic meaning.

As many psychomotor phenomena are treated in the recent literature, restlessness, conceptualized interchangeably with "psychomotor agitation,"[10] is also considered by many scientists in the context of neuropsychophysiological explanations. Olds (1976) postulates the effects of catecholamines on agitation, especially psychotic agitation, and many recent studies of amines' effects on behaviors have attributed restlessness as the effects of cimetidine or amphetamines. In addition, nocturnal restlessness of cardiac patients has been explained as the hypoxic response in several recent studies; such explanations might suggest relationships among cerebral hypoxia, catecholamine release, motor activities, and apprehension.

While it is not too difficult to recognize a person in a state of restlessness, restlessness is difficult to define explicitly for several reasons. First, it is often used to indicate a state of mind, as in "I am restless. The spring air must be affecting me!" even though the person may not exhibit behaviors of restlessness. Second, it is also often used to describe behaviors objectively observed, as in "He is restless today; he acts likes a tiger in a cage." Third, it can be a fleeting or long-lasting experiential phenomenon in which many different kinds of body and motor movements are possible. And fourth, historically it has been described as one aspect of more complex phenomena, such as schizophrenia, depression, anxiety, fear, hyperthyroidism, hypoglycemia, and dysphoria.

Furthermore, it has seldom been treated in scientific fields as a distinct phenomenon. The phenomenon of restlessness, it seems, should be conceptualized with respect to the nature of motor activity and the associated feeling state. Therefore, restlessness may be tentatively defined as a state in which a person exhibits purposeless and irrepressible body movements and activities accompanied with a feeling of tension and uneasiness.

## Differentiation of the Concept from Anxiety and Fear

The major aspect that differentiates restlessness from anxiety and fear is the emphasis on motor activities and the specificity of the feeling state. While all three concepts deal with phenomena that occur in persons in stressful, emotional states, accompanied with neurophysiological and motor behaviors, restlessness as a concept is confined to phenomena in which specific kinds of motor activities are exhibited with a feeling state of uneasiness. In contrast, anxiety refers primarily to a state of an emotion that is subjectively felt and consciously perceived tension, apprehension, and nervousness. It is usually accompanied by or associated with activation of the autonomic nervous system (Speilberger, 1975). Anxiety may be expressed in many behavioral forms, including restless motor activities. Thus, restlessness as a concept may be considered an element in a more general class of phenomena called "anxiety."

The concept of fear is less similar to the concept of restlessness, but it is possible to imagine the presence of restless behaviors when a person is in a state of mild fear. In general, fear refers to an emotional state in which a person feels the possible, pending imposition of an undesirable, noxious, dangerous, or threatening condition. It is expressed in various behavioral forms through the activation of the autonomic nervous system, ranging from a total frozen state to a frantic flight. The emotional state of fear is focused and usually has a specific object by which fearful emotions are elicited. In these respects, the phenomenon of restlessness differs from fear more definitely than the phenomenon differs from anxiety.

## Operationalization

Very little work is available in the literature on the operationalization of the concept of restlessness. Many descriptions of restlessness have been used by nurses in clinical situations; many are subjectively derived understandings of restless behaviors. Norris describes restlessness as the following:

> Restlessness seems to be expressed in many ways: by tossing, turning, or twisting in bed, by pacing, tapping with fingers or feet, picking with the fingers, scratching, or other motor activity of a repetitive, seemingly urgent, and not purposefully controlled or directed nature. Facial expressions may be tense, watchful, or fearful. The rate or amount of speech may increase.[11]

Clinical manifestations of restlessness appear to be irregular and are subject to personal interpretations. The common procedure used in studies is usually descriptive in nature and is indicated by a gross measure of judgment for the degree or presence of agitated motor movements.

Since an operationalization of a concept depends on the explicit definition of the concept adopted or developed, we assume that this operationalization, given the definition advanced above, requires at least two dimensional measurements: (a) the nature of motor activity, and (b) feeling state. There are several characteristics inherent in the restless motor activity—aimlessness of movements, irrepressibility of movements, and fussiness of movements. In addition, an accompanying feeling state of generalized tension, uneasiness, nonspecific distress, irritability, or belligerence needs to be included in the measurement strategies to express the phenomenon of restlessness.

Duration is also suggestive of an important aspect of restlessness, manifested clinically in patient-care situations. Intensity of restlessness is another aspect of clinical manifestation requiring nursing attention, yet there seems to be no objective way of differentiating degrees of intensity. At best, the measure of restlessness has to be descriptive with respect to motor activities and movements. Measurement of restlessness for the dimension of the feeling state is problematic, since it has to depend upon the client's expressions of feelings.

### Relationships with Other Concepts

There is a paucity of research that deals specifically with restlessness in patients. Few studies in the literature deal with the hypoxia hypothesis, which suggests that restless behaviors may be the responses to hypoxia. Restlessness also has been considered the response to cerebral anoxia, usually resulting from injury. Norris (1975) alludes to several possible causes of restlessness, such as changes in the rhythmicity of life, anticipation of change, fatigue and boredom, role-deprivation, as well as many pathophysiological conditions.

Conceptualization of restlessness in a global, experiential sense is not found in the literature. Clinical observations and experiences suggest that restlessness is related to such experiences of hospitalized patients as unfamiliarity of surroundings, stress of illness or surgery, symbolic and physical meanings of isolation, and altered perceptions. A better understanding of restlessness-inducing factors within the person, the environment, and in experiences can help develop nursing interventions that can be applied to clients who become restless. There may be many experiential and symbolic factors as well as physical ones in hospitalization and illness experiences that tend to arouse restlessness in certain clients. In addition, studies differentiating psychotic/schizophrenic agitation and simple restlessness should be of interest for a better understanding of neuropsychophysiological propositions, especially those related to catecholamine physiology.

## COMPLIANCE

- A bottle full of antihypertensive drug on the night stand having the prescription filling date six months old.
- Four plus sugar of a diabetic client's urine test for the past four consecutive visits to the nurse practitioner at a clinic.
- Missed clinic visits by a patient on cardiac medication.
- Two packs of cigarettes smoked daily by a client who has an advanced chronic obstructive lung disease and bronchial asthma.
- A 3,000 calorie diet consumed repeatedly by a client on a 1,000 calorie reducing-diet regime.

## Definition

These are but a few examples of noncompliance in health care, as expressed in the literature. At the conclusion of the Workshop/Symposium on Compliance with Therapeutic Regimens at McMaster University held in May 1974, the group accepted a general definition of *compliance* as *the extent to which the patient's behavior coincides with the clinical prescription* (Sackett, 1976). In contrast to this definition of compliance, which is suggestive of the neutrality of the concept, there have been many definitions of compliance suggested by health-care practitioners and scholars that encompass the notion of power influence on the behaviors of conformity. Barofsky (1978) attaches coercion to the phenomenon of compliance, maintaining the negative meaning of the concept. Because of this, compliance raises an ethical issue dealing with client autonomy. The negative connotation of the term has been the focus of many debates among physicians, nurses, behavioral and social scientists, and social workers.

The primary difference between the definitions proposed by the Sackett group and by Barofsky can be found in the perspectives from which the phenomena are conceptualized. The first approach in which alignment of client's behaviors with prescriptions as a definition of compliance views the phenomena as a property concept. Here, the notion of how compliant behaviors may result is removed from the definition, and it only refers to the client's behaviors judged against the clinical prescriptions for adherence and conformity. Thus, in the health-care field, compliance as a property concept has an accepted meaning that refers to the adherence and coincidence of a client's behaviors to professional prescriptions.

In contrast, compliance as a process concept refers to the client's behaviors that vary according to the degree with which others influence the behaviors (Barofsky, 1978). This form of definition depicts the process of influence in which power to influence is exercised to produce certain behaviors in the client. Thus, characteristically, the same client behaviors (i.e., by an objective judgment, such as taking medication at certain hours of the day, or making return clinic visits faithfully) may be classified as compliance, adherence, or therapeutic alliance, depending upon whether the behavior is produced by (a) coercion that is thought to produce *compliance,* (b) conformity that is thought to result in *adherence,* or (c) negotiation that is considered to bring about *therapeutic alliance.* For this definition of the concept, what is central to the phenomenon is not the nature of behaviors exhibited by the client but the way the behaviors are induced from the client. That is, it is important to differentiate whether the behaviors are produced by coercive pressure, self-propelled conformity, or negotiation between the client and the professional in which some type of transaction occurs. It is theoretically important because an understanding of such processes is necessary for predicting future behaviors.

In conceptualizing the phenomenon of compliance, there also has been some debate about what should constitute "clinical prescriptions." Medication orders, return visits, dietary modifications, exercise programs, curtailment of smoking, abstinance of alcoholic consumption, and other changes in personal habits have been included as examples of clinical prescriptions in the field. Since the phenomenon of compliance refers to self-administered regimens without the constant surveillance by professional staff that exists in institutionalized care settings, clinical prescriptions generally refer to the kinds of activities and modifications of behaviors related to daily habits. The object is development of new behavioral patterns or modifications of existing ones. These behaviors are usually in the core of the client's private life.

Sackett (1976) introduces the intended goal, in terms of prevention, management, and rehabilitation, as an additional dimension of the clinical prescriptions. He shows that the studies reviewed suggest different levels of compliance, not only according to the types of regimen but also according to the intended goals of regimen.

This diversity in conceptualization of compliance suggests the complexity of the behavioral patterns linked to compliance, and begs for a unified theory of compliance.

## Operationalization

Expression of compliance in measurable terms has been the major difficulty for the researchers in the field. Although there have been many studies using various types of direct or indirect measures of compliance, there is no consensus as to what would explicitly and accurately reflect the degree of compliance. Gordis (1976) surveyed many studies of compliance and found that there is neither a general agreement on the definition that distinguishes compliance from noncompliance, nor is there a measurement system that expresses the true meaning of compliance in terms of outcome. Direct measures, such as the rate of drug excretion and blood levels of drugs, to test the compliance to medication-taking has been found to be more reliable than pill-counting or self-reporting. However, it has been suspected that explanations of compliance may be masked by measurement errors in both types of methods.

Many of the indirect measures that use outcomes of regimens as the criteria for compliance, such as blood pressure level, weight-reduction rate, or respiratory capacity, have been found to be influenced by many other physiological and transient variables as well as regimen-compliance. In many instances, such measurements tend to yield minimal information about compliance.

Another major operationalization problem is in the comparability of compliance to one regimen with that to another. For example, there is no conceptual or operational clarity in handling the similarities and differences between compliance to a hypertensive medication and compliance to a low-salt diet. Obviously, the motivational and behavioral constraints that influence compliance to these two regimens are quite different. The complex nature of clinical prescriptions and the requirements these pose on individuals remain to be the most critical aspect of the phenomenon of compliance both theoretically and operationally.

Measurement of compliance relying on self-reporting has received a great deal of criticism for its reliability as well. Many studies found discrepancies between what clients report and their actual behaviors, although there continue to be reports of compliance studies using this form of operationalization, for the lack of a better or more convenient measure.

### Relationships with Other Concepts

Compliance literature abounds with research studies that link compliance with different concepts in the domain of client, such as motivation, amount of knowledge, cognitive dissonance, and the presence of serious symptoms. The health-belief model (Becker, 1974) has been used in many studies as the theoretical framework, trying to explain compliance on the basis of clients' internal states and definitions of situations. These explanations are mainly oriented to treating compliance as an essentially self-triggered phenomenon. Thus, compliance is viewed as a behavioral outcome of other personal traits and characteristics, such as (a) how motivated a person is to attain a healthy state, (b) how much a certain state of health is valued by the person, (c) what the extent is to which a person believes his or her conduct will result in a positive outcome, (d) what the extent is for a person to maintain a cognitively conflicting situation, and (e) how much a person knows about the nature of illness and the effectiveness of treatment.

In addition, several concepts in the domain of environment, such as social support, social pressure, and symbolic expectations, also have been found to have influence on a client's compliance. In the domain of nursing action, characteristics of client-nurse interaction, contracting, and collaborative decision-making have also been studied to explain compliance in the client. The degree to which a client receives reinforcement, positive feedback, frequent support or supportive knowledge generated by the client's interactions with significant others and professionals, as well as the degree to which a client receives pressure for conformity have been shown to influence compliance with various types of clinical prescriptions.

Hence, it suggests that compliance is related to influences of internal and external types as seen from the perspective of the client. The exact nature of the processes by which both internal and external factors mediate compliance has not been studied extensively and needs to be investigated.


## SUMMARY

Since this chapter contains a great deal of new terminology and several new ideas in conceptualization, it is perhaps worthwhile to point out the main ideas that have been discussed. The domain of client as the focus of conceptualization is shown to contain diverse types of concepts and phenomena essential for theoretical thinking in nursing.

It appears that rethinking of the models of man and health is central to clarifying both philosophical and theoretical stances that are necessary for theoretical thinkers to assume in nursing. It might be useful to examine many and varied models of man and health that are currently used as the basis for theoretical developments in other scientific fields in order to attain a greater clarity in the theoretical requirements for nursing models of man and health. It also seems fruitful to reexamine nursing models of man and health that are being used in research and practice for their theoretical breadth and limitations.

While there are many different ways of categorizing concepts in the domain of client for studies from the nursing perspective, the suggested typology of essentialistic, developmental, problematic, and health-care experiential types provides a beginning for examining the conceptual properties in a systematic way. By way of examples, attempts are made to show how to ask important questions in definitional clarification of concept, operationalization of concept, and in considering relationships of concept with other related phenomena. Restlessness and compliance were discussed to show the use of these strategies in conceptual analysis.

The main thrust in conceptualization for the domain of client is in developing, ultimately, a nursing theory of humanity or a nursing theory of health that can be the basis for understanding a diverse array of problems presented by the client whom we encounter in nursing. In addition, the need for development of middle range theories aimed at understanding boundary-specific phenomena in clients has been implicitly stressed in the discussions of restlessness and compliance. Middle range theories in nursing that deal with broad, particularistic phenomena in the domain of client will help us accumulate the many layers of theoretical knowledge necessary for a development of grand nursing theories.

## BIBLIOGRAPHY

Ahmed, PI, and Coelho, GV (eds.). *Toward a New Definition of Health: Psychosocial Dimensions.* New York: Plenum Press, 1979

Balis, GM, Wurmser, L, and McDaniel, E (eds.). *The Behavioral and Social Sciences and the Practice of Medicine.* Boston: Butterworth Publishers, 1978

Bandura, A. *Principles of Behavior Modification.* New York: Holt, Reinhardt, and Winston, 1969

Barnes, R, and Murray, R. Strategies for Diagnosing and Treating Agitation in the Aging. *Geriatrics* 35: 111–119, 1980

Barofsky, I. Compliance, Adherence, and the Therapeutic Alliance: Steps in the Development of Self-Care. *Soc Sci Med* 12A: 369–376, 1978

Barrett, W. *The Illusion of Technique.* Garden City, NY: Anchor Press, 1978

Becker, MH. The Health Belief Model and Personal Health Behavior. *Health Educ Monogr* 2: 326–473, 1974

Becker, MH. Sociobehavioral Determinants of Compliance. In DL Sackett and RB Haynes (eds.): *Compliance with Therapeutic Regimens.* Baltimore: The Johns Hopkins University Press, 1976, pp 40–50

Blau, PM (ed.). *Approaches to the Study of Social Structure.* New York: The Free Press, 1975

Blazer, D, and Williams, C. Epidemiology of Dysphoria and Depression in an Elderly Population. *Am J Psychiatry* 137: 439–444, 1980

Breslow, L. A Quantitative Approach to the WHO Definition of Health. *Int J Epidemiol* 1: 287–294; 347–355, 1972

Brook, RH, Ware, JE, Davis-Avery, A, et al. Overview of Adult Health Status Measures Fielded in Rand's Health Insurance Study. *Med Care* (Supplement) 17: 1–131, 1979

Brown, NO. *Life Against Death: The Psychoanalytical Meaning of History.* Wesleyan: Wesleyan University Press, 1959

Browning, DS. *Generative Man: Psychoanalytic Perspectives.* Philadelphia: The Westminster Press, 1973

Cannon, WB. *The Wisdom of the Body.* New York: W.W. Norton, 1932

Clark, AR, et al. Lower Limit on Neutral-Heavy Muon Mass. *Phys Rev Letters* 46: 299–302, 1981

Dobzhansky, T. *The Biology of Ultimate Concern.* New York: The New American Library, 1967

Dubos, R. *Man Adapting.* New Haven: Yale University Press, 1965

Dubos, R. The State of Health and the Quality of Life. *West J Med* 125: 8–11, 1976

Engel, GL. Sudden Death and the Medical Model in Psychiatry. *Can Psychiatr Assoc J* 15: 527–538, 1970

Engel, GL. A Unified Concept of Health and Disease. In T Mullin (ed.): *Medical Behavioral Science.* Philadelphia: W.B. Saunders, 1975, pp 185–200

Engelhardt, HT, Jr. Ideology and Etiology. *J Med Philos* 1: 256–268, 1976

English, HB, and English, AC. *A Comprehensive Dictionary of Psychological and Psychoanalytical Terms.* New York: Longman, Green, 1958

Erde, EL. Mind-Body and Malady. *J Med Philos* 2: 177–190, 1977

Erde, EL. Philosophical Considerations Regarding Defining ''Health,'' ''Disease,'' etc., and Their Bearing on Medical Practice. *Ethics Sci Med* 6: 31–48, 1978

Erikson, EH. *Identity and the Life Cycle: Selected Papers.* Psychological Issues Monograph, Vol.1, no.1. New York: International University Press, 1959

Erikson, EH. *Insight and Responsibility: Lectures on the Ethical Implications of Psychoanalytic Insight.* New York: W.W. Norton, 1964

Fabrega, H, Jr. *Disease and Social Behavior: An Interdisciplinary Perspective.* Cambridge: MIT Press, 1974

Fabrega, H. The Position of Psychiatric Illness in Biomedical Theory: A Cultural Analysis. *J Med Philos* 5: 145–168, 1980

Fauman, MA. Treatment of the Agitated Patient with an Organic Brain Disorder. *JAMA* 240: 380–382, 1978

Fletcher, J. *Humanhood: Essays in Biomedical Ethics.* Buffalo, NY: Prometheus Books, 1979

Fromm, E. *Man for Himself.* New York: Rinehart Company, 1947

Fromm, E. *The Heart of Man: Its Genesis for Good and Evil.* New York: Harper and Row, 1964

Fromm, E, and Xiran, R (eds.). *The Nature of Man: A Reader.* New York: Macmillan, 1968

Garrity, TF, Somes, GW, and Marx, MB. Factors Influencing Self-Assessment of Health. *Soc Sci Med* 12A: 77–81, 1978

Given, CW, Simoni, L, and Gallin, R. The Design and Use of a Health Status Index for Family Physician. *J Fam Pract* 4: 287–291, 1977

Goldberg, WG, and Fitzpatrick, JJ. Movement Therapy with the Aged. *Nurs Res* 29: 339–346, 1980

Gordis, L. Methodologic Issues in the Measurement of Patient Compliance. In DL Sackett and RB Haynes (eds.): *Compliance with Therapeutic Regimens.* Baltimore: The Johns Hopkins University Press, 1976, pp 51–66

Hartman, H. *Ego Psychology and the Problems of Adaptation,* Trans. by David Rapoport. New York: International Universities Press, 1958

Haynes, RB. A Critical Review of the ''Determinants'' of Patient Compliance with Therapeutic Regimen. In DL Sackett and RB Haynes (eds.): *Compliance with Therapeutic Regimens.* Baltimore: The Johns Hopkins University Press, 1976, pp 26–39

Helson, HH. *Adaptation Level Theory.* New York: Harper & Row, 1956

Hinkle, LE. Ecological Observations of the Relation of Physical Illness, Mental Illness, and the Social Environment. *Psychosom Med* 23: 289–297, 1961

Homans, GC. *Social Behavior: Its Elementary Forms.* New York: Harcourt, Brace, 1961

Howard, H, and Scott, RA. Proposed Framework for the Analysis of Stress in the Human Organism. *Behav Sci* 10: 141–160, 1965

Hull, CL. *Essentials of Behavior.* New Haven: Yale University Press, 1951

Hunt, SM, and McEwen, J. The Development of a Subjective Health Indicator. *Social Health Illness* 2: 231–246, 1980

Johnson, DE. *The Behavioral System Model for Nursing.* A Paper Presented at the University of Delaware. Newark, Delaware: June 14, 1977

Johnson, DE. The Behavioral System Model for Nursing. In SC Roy and JP Riehl (eds.): *Conceptual Models for Nursing Practice,* Second edition. New York: Appleton-Century-Crofts, 1980

Kaplan, RM, Bush, JW, and Berry, CC. Health Status: Types of Validity and the Index of Well-being. *Health Serv Res* 11: 478–507, 1976

Kelman, S. Social Organization and the Meaning of Health. *J Med Philos* 5: 133–144, 1980

Kennedy, LW, Northcott, HC, and Kinzel, C. Subjective Evaluation of Well-being: Problems and Prospects. *Soc Indicators Res* 5: 457–474, 1978

Keyser, CJ. *Mathematical Philosophy.* New York: E.P. Dutton, 1924

Korzybski, A. *Manhood of Humanity.* New York: E.P. Dutton, 1921

Kunkel, J, and Nagasawa, RH. A Behavioral Model of Man: Propositions and Implications. *Am Sociol Rev* 38: 530–543, 1973

Maddox, GL. Self-Assessment of Health Status. *J Chronic Dis* 17: 449, 1964

Maslow, AH. A Theory of Metamotivation: The Biological Rooting of the Value-Life. *J Human Psychol* 7: 93–127, 1967

Maslow, AH. Towards a Humanistic Biology. In J Stulman and E Laszlo (eds.): *Emergent Man: His Chances, Problems and Potentials.* New York: Gordon and Breach, 1973, pp 1–23

Moos, RH. *The Human Context: Environmental Determinants of Behavior.* New York: Wiley Interscience, 1976

Moravcsik, J. Ancient and Modern Conceptions of Health and Medicine. *J Med Philos* 1: 337, 1976

Mushkin, SJ, and Dunlop, DW (eds.). *Health: What Is It Worth? Measures of Health Benefits.* New York: Pergamon Press, 1979

Naegel, KD. *Health and Healing.* Compiled and Edited by E. Cummings. San Francisco: Jossey-Bass, 1970

Newman, MA. *Theory Development in Nursing.* Philadelphia: F.A. Davis, 1979

Norris, CM. Restlessness: A Nursing Phenomenon in Search of Meaning. *Nurs Outlook* 23: 103–107, 1975

Nursing Theories Conference Group. *Nursing Theories: The Base for Professional Nursing Practice.* Englewood Cliffs, NJ: Prentice-Hall, 1980

Olds, J. Behavioral Studies of Hypothalamic Functions: Drives and Reinforcements. In RG Grennell and S Gagay (eds.): *Biological Foundations of Psychiatry.* New York: Raven Press, 1976

Orem, DE. *Nursing: Concepts of Practice,* Second edition. New York: McGraw-Hill, 1980

Parsons, T. *The Social System.* New York: The Free Press, 1951

Parsons, T. The Definitions of Health and Illness in the Light of American Values and Social Structure. In GE Jaco (ed.): *Patients, Physicians, and Illness.* Glenco, IL: The Free Press, 1958

Pennington, JE, and Mask, EJ. Case-Record of the Massachusetts General Hospital: Case 28–1980—Pneumonia in a 62 Year Old Man with Chronic Lymphocytic Leukemia. *N Engl J Med* 303: 145–152, 1980

Polakov, WN. *Man and His Affairs: From the Engineering Point of View.* Baltimore: Williams and Wilkins, 1925

Redlick, FC. Editorial Reflections on the Concepts of Health and Disease. *J Med Philos* 1: 269–280, 1976

Rieff, P. *Freud: The Mind of the Moralist.* New York: Doubleday, 1961

Rieff, P. *The Triumph of the Therapeutics: Uses of Faith after Freud.* New York: Harper and Row, 1966

Rogers, ME. *An Introduction to the Theoretical Basis of Nursing.* Philadelphia: F.A. Davis, 1970

Rogers, ME. Nursing: A Science of Unitary Man. In SC Roy and JP Riehl (eds.): *Concep-*

*tual Models for Nursing Practice,* Second edition. New York: Appleton-Century-Crofts, 1980, pp 329–337

Roy, SC. Adaptation: A Conceptual Framework for Nursing. *Nurs Outlook* 18: 42–45, 1970

Roy, SC. *Introduction to Nursing: An Adaptation Model.* Englewood Cliffs, NJ: Prentice-Hall, 1976

Roy, SC, and Riehl, JP. *Conceptual Models for Nursing Practice,* Second edition. New York: Appleton-Century-Crofts, 1980

Roy, SC, and Roberts, SL. *Theory Construction in Nursing: An Adaptation Model.* Englewood Cliffs, NJ: Prentice-Hall, 1981

Royce, JE. *Man and His Nature: A Philosophical Psychology.* New York: McGraw-Hill, 1961

Sackett, DL. Introduction and the Magnitude of Compliance and Noncompliance. In DL Sackett and RB Haynes (eds.): *Compliance with Therapeutic Regimens.* Baltimore: The Johns Hopkins University Press, 1976, pp 1–25

Selye, H. *The Stress of Life.* New York: McGraw-Hill, 1956

Selye, H. *The Stress of Life,* Revised edition. New York: McGraw-Hill, 1976

Simon, H. *Models of Man.* New York: John Wiley, 1957

Simon, H. *Models of Thoughts.* New Haven: Yale University Press, 1979

Skinner, BF. *Science and Human Behavior.* New York: Macmillan, 1953

Smith, JA. The Idea of Health: A Philosophical Inquiry. *Adv Nurs Sci* 3: 43–50, 1981

Sontag, S. *Illness as Metaphor.* New York: Farrar, Straus, and Giroux, 1977

Spielberger, CD. Anxiety: State-Trait-Process? In CD Spielberger and IG Sarasen (eds.): *Stress and Anxiety,* Vol.1. Washington, DC: Hemisphere, 1975

Turnbull, A. Measurement of Health. *Am J Nurs* 76: 1985–1987, 1976

Twaddle, AC. The Concept of Health Status. *Soc Sci Med* 8: 29–38, 1974

Wan, T. Predicting Self-Assessed Health Status: A Multivariate Approach. *Health Serv Res* 11: 464–477, 1976

Wolff, HG. A Concept of Disease in Man. *Psychosom Med* 24: 25–30, 1962

Woody, RH (ed.). *Encyclopedia of Clinical Assessment,* Vols. 1 and 2. San Francisco: Jossey-Bass, 1980

Zola, IK. Culture and Symptoms: An Analysis of Patients' Presenting Complaints. *Am Sociol Rev* 31: 615–630, 1966

# 5

# Theoretical Analysis of Phenomena in the Domain of Environment

... the man of flesh, bone, and illusions will always experience unexpected difficulties as he tries to adapt to the real world, which is often hostile to him.

*René Dubos*

## OVERVIEW

In the preceding chapter, the theoretical nature of phenomena in humans is examined within the nursing perspective. The purpose of this chapter is to shift the focus to human environment, and examine the relevance of environmental factors in a consideration of human health and nursing practice. The fundamental question for the purpose of this chapter is: In what ways and to what extent is it useful to analyze environment from the nursing perspective? This chapter deals with this question in three steps. In the first section, delineation of the general characteristics of the domain of environment is carried out, paying attention to spatial, temporal, and qualitative meanings of environmental elements. Expositions also deal with essential aspects of environment with reference to client and nursing practice. In addition, the holistic approach to conceptualization of human environment, especially that advocated by Rogers (1970 and 1980), is examined for its theoretical and methodological adequacies.

In the second section, each qualitative component of environment, categorized as *physical, social,* and *symbolic* environment, is analyzed theoretically. Distinct bodies of knowledge and specific theoretical perspectives exist for each component, making separate expositions helpful.

Three concepts (sensory deprivation, social support, and sick-role expectation) selected from each component of environment are analyzed in the next section as the illustrations of conceptual analysis applied to the domain of environment. These analyses show different ways of conceptualizing selected aspects of environment and how such conceptualizations are linked to different phenomena in nursing. Relationships between these selected concepts from the domain of environment and several important phenomena in the domain of client are examined in this section as well. The aim is to show the extent to which explanations of human phenomena may be attributed to environmental factors from the nursing perspective.

## THE DOMAIN OF ENVIRONMENT

Human living is carried on in a changing context that we call environment. Our feet rest on the ground that is a part of the planet Earth because we are unable to float about in the air; we breathe the air, that of varying degrees of cleanliness; we sometimes are able to claim many acres of land as ours, but we are sometimes forced to occupy only several cubic feet of space for our body; we can see a setting sun and feel pleasantly affected by its beauty, or depressed by the burden of a lost day; we pray to God for salvation, but we at other times participate in a dance to chase away demons; and we wake up in the morning next to a loving person, as we at other times run away from our parents, friends, or enemies in desperation. And such factors cause us to be malnourished or fat, to have goiter or scurvy, to be healthy or sick, to be lonely or content, and to feel secure or anxious. Environment is the essential part of human existence.

Environment is defined as the entity that exists external to a person or to humanity, conceived either as a whole or as that containing many distinct elements. Thus, this definition does not include what Bernard called *milieu interieur* as a part of environment. A person's functioning and development are partly constrained and determined by the nature of the environment in which the person finds or positions himself or herself. Many human health conditions have been found to be associated with environmental factors. For example, regional differences have been found in studies of the prevalence of dental caries (Ludwig, 1968). Effects of ecology on nutritional stress (Newman, 1968), black lung diseases among miners, and neurosis in industrial societies highlight the effects of environment on people's health. Feibleman delineates the relationship between human nature and the environment, in a spirit similar to Dobzhansky's (1962) and Dubos' (1965) espousal of the environmental control of human conditions:

> Where he [man] begins is determined by the equipment he brings with him to his birth, and it is considerable. He inherits the past of his ancestors, and thus acquires all sorts of capabilities and limitations; but he acquires during infancy the responses to artifactual [tool and language] and social stimuli. He is in contact with tools from the cradle, and adults make signs to him in it.[1]

Yet, it does not suffice to say only that human conditions and experiences such as health, illness, happiness, or growth are affected by the environment. It is necessary to go one step further and consider that human nature also allows conscious and purposeful use of environmental conditions for the benefit of existence. Control of environment has been one of the many persisting human preoccupations, especially that of Western humanity. Modern civilization and technology, specifically, suggest the advances people have made in controlling their environment. People have created changes in their environment over its history, and likewise have been affected by the changes.

Recent demonstrations by people in Europe and America against the proliferation of nuclear weapons and demonstrations in various sites in the U.S. against the construction of nuclear power plants, as well as the incident of Three-Mile Island, suggest our concern regarding the influence and the potential influence of a "created" environment on human life. At the same time, factors in a person's more immediate environment, such as crowding or pollution, can be attributed to having an influence on the person's state of health, growth, and feelings. In a strict sense, human existence cannot be considered out of environmental context.

For our analysis, this context, i.e., environment, is considered in terms of three characteristics making a complex entity: (a) *spatial*, (b) *temporal*, and (c) *qualitative*. These three characteristics of environment provide different frameworks for conceptualizing environment. Environment in a spatial sense is conceptualized in concentric circles around the person in the center, indicating proximity of environmental elements to the person. Spatial aspects of the environment also circumscribe the size of its boundary. Thus, if we consider the universe as the total environment of a person, some of its elements are parts of the immediate milieu, located within the inner ring. Such elements in the immediate environment have a rather direct impact upon a person's life. On the other hand, many elements are remote, existing in the outer circles. Such elements influence the person only in marginal ways. Yet all elements in the environment in totality represent a context within which one lives.

Temporally defined environment, on the other hand, encompasses aspects of environment with respect to duration and manner of presence. Hence we may have environments of which elements exist (a) continuously, intermittently, or fleetingly, and (b) regularly or randomly. The first characteristic of the presence of elements in the environment is related to duration and is suggestive of permanence and temporariness. The second characteristic (regularly or randomly) is related to the manner of presence, that is, whether elements exist in the environment in a patterned, systematic way, or in a haphazard, irregular manner. Whether or not an environmental element is present in one's surroundings rather permanently will determine to a certain degree the amount of its influence on a person, although certainly the element's quality will affect the degree of its influence.

The third way of conceptualizing environment focuses on the qualitative aspect of the environmental elements, thought of in terms of *physical, social,* and *symbolic* qualities. Accordingly, environment can be classified into three subenvironments—physical environment, social environment, and symbolic environment—by dividing the environmental elements by their characteristics in these three respects. This differentiation is similar to the conceptualization offered by Murdock (1980) in which he distinguishes physical, social, and ideational environment. Parsons' notion (1951) of the object world of an individual, which is thought to be composed of physical, social, and cultural objects, is also akin to this categorization. Parsons defines the object world as a situation of social interaction in which physical objects are means and conditions of one's actions, social objects provide specific orientations of interaction, and cultural objects provide symbolic elements for definition of interaction (Parsons, 1951). For our conceptualization, the object world, i.e., environment, is considered not only for situations of social interaction but also for situations of human living of all sorts.

Physical environment consists of the energy-generating, matter-based aspects of milieu that are in various forms of biotic and abiotic elements. Social environment, on the other hand, refers to individuals and groups with whom a person interacts and communicates. Family members, friends, colleagues, neighbors, and other people who may be remotely placed constitute one's social environment. In contrast to these two categories of environment (physical and social), which are more concretely based in the empirical world and are in concrete forms, symbolic environment consists of (a) ideational elements such as ideas, values, beliefs, and knowledge; (b) normative elements such as rules, laws, expectations, and constraints; and (c) institutional elements such as roles, organizations, institutions, society, and culture. These are elements that have no physical or concrete forms and exist only in people's minds. The symbolic environment is the specific artifact of human history, in that contents of the symbolic environment are the products of life stories of anonymous successions of ancestors and contemporaries.

Figure 3 shows the relationships among the three aspects describing and defining an environment, and suggests variability in its compositions in three dimensions. Contracting and expanding natures of the three components, namely physical, social, and symbolic components, depicted in Time 1 and Time 2 sequences are characterized by spatiality and by temporal effects that change the

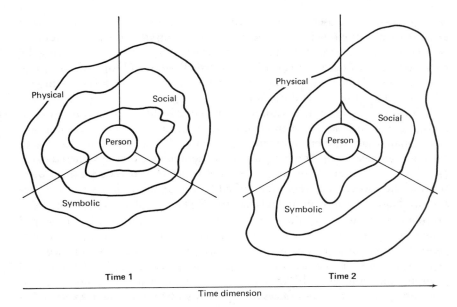

*Figure 3.* Aspects of client's environment—time, space, components (physical, social, and symbolic).

manners with which the qualitative constituents of the environment are present in it.

The concept of environment proposed here implies that environment can be perceived either as a whole, encompassing the totality in the three dimensions, or as separated spheres of milieu viewed according to size (spatiality), continuity (temporality), or constituents (qualitative components). Specifically, the three dimensional differentiations pose possible variability in an environment. For example, an environment can be indicated as a specific physical territory containing physical elements that stay or disappear randomly, or as a vast symbolic and social field such as a scientific community.

Inherent in these ways of conceptualizing human environment is the idea that elements of the environment are perceived by the person through the senses and are evaluated according to the affective and cognitive structures developed within the person. Therefore, sensory perception is the basis of knowing what exists, while cognitive and affective evaluation allows the person to attach meanings to whatever is perceived to exist. Hence we like the setting sun, interpret a touch as caressing, etc. However, there are elements in the environment that are not perceived consciously, nor evaluated to have a specific meaning. Such elements may nevertheless exert influences on one's life.

Then, what are useful ways of examining environment and phenomena of environment in the nursing perspective? The nursing perspective requires conceptualization of environment in two specific ways: (a) environment having the client as an individual at the core of the concentric field; and (b) environment as nursing care environment in which the environment takes one specific symbolic meaning, that of health and nursing.

For the first concern, environment of client is the external reality that is identifiable according to the three dimensions proposed in the preceding section. Analytically, the environment of the client needs to be considered with specific references to his or her health. This orientation is basically related to examining Dubos' proposition that "the states of health or disease are the expressions of the success or failure experienced by the organism in its efforts to respond adaptively to environmental changes."[2] Theoretical interests, then, are in extracting those aspects of the client's environment (or human environment in general) that are more closely tied to human conditions of health. Dubos (1965) views the environment as physical, biological, and social forces and qualities, and defines health in terms of a person functioning in a given physical and social environment. Inherent in his notion is the idea that environment not only provides the circumstances and forces for a person's adaptation that is expressed as health, but is also a context in which health as "functioning" is defined for the individual. The environment is taken as a whole in which a person acts, reacts, and interacts within the confines of genotypic and phenotypic givens and of the potentialities of self-determination, and through which one occupies changing states of health.

Rogers (1970 and 1980) conceptualizes the environment in a holistic way, although her approach is more totally unitary than that postulated by Dubos. Dubos (1965) maintains the separateness of different components of the environment in his analysis of the specific effects of different environmental forces on human condition. Rogers views environment as one open system that should be considered in its totality as an energy field (1970). Rogers' conceptualization of environment may be best understood within the current physics' world view, the theory of relativity. Einstein's general theory of relativity suggests that the universe as a construct of space, in a relativistic sense, is curved, and that the flow of time in that universe is "relative" to the timekeeper's state of motion. Since this assumption holds for the general case, that is, with a holistic world view, and is tied to the notion of dematerialization of matter into energy (i.e., matter as concentrated patterns of energy), environment in this view is a spatial, temporal entity consisting of energy patterns.

Accordingly, Rogers proposes that the universe is an energy field within which the human field and its environmental field coexist only in a relativistic sense. Environment is conceptualized as "a four dimensional, negentropic energy field identified by pattern and organization, and encompassing all that are outside any given human field" (Rogers, 1980, p. 332). It is also considered to be unique to each human person. To Rogers, environment is that possessing a spatial and temporal boundary, and expressed as a patterned and organized field of energy. It is seen as a totality, an entity that is only expressible as a whole. Therefore, to Rogers, environment is a variable only in terms of energy of pattern and organization.

Operationalization of this conceptualization has been found wanting, because the energizing phenomena of an environmental field as the manifestations of the totality are empirically difficult to grasp for understanding as well as for measuring. However, Rogers' global posture of conceptualizing environment may be a fruitful way of looking at the world, especially if we are interested in considering human health in a holistic manner. According to Rogers' model, nurses and nursing actions as elements of the external world of a client are imperceptible, totally interfused aspects of the environment. The environment as a totality is represented as an energy field, having certain kinds of patterns and organization. What is rather confusing in Rogers' conceptualization of environment is her conceptualization that both human and environmental systems are expressed as energy fields. Possible differences in the characteristics of energy fields have not been clearly conceptualized. For instance, the human energy field is alluded to be more complex because of human consciousness and creativity, yet the exact nature of that complexity and its difference from the environmental energy field, which is composed of both animate and inanimate elements, is not specified in the model. Specifying similarities and differences between the human field and the environmental field will give a greater explanatory credence.

Other nursing theorists view environment in a rather casual manner. King (1981), for example, conceptualizes environment as the world that is perceived by a person, composed of people and things that are sources of stressors for the person. This view is useful insofar as it is adopted in the interactional contexts with which King is mainly concerned. In a similar fashion, theorists such as Neuman (1980), Roy (1980), and others having a theoretical orientation in systems models of stress/adaptation also view environment as that from which stresses and stimulations are generated to the individual and with which the individual tries to attain balance. The exact nature of environment and the mechanisms by which stresses originate in the environment are neither defined nor explored in these models. For such conceptualization, nurses and nursing actions are capable of generating stresses and stimulations to the client as parts of the environment.

A nursing environment can be conceived as that specifically defined in social terms, in which a person becomes designated as a client. A nursing environment evolves around this client who is the recipient of nursing services from others who have been designated as nursing care givers. In a nursing environment, spatial and qualitative characteristics are different from the person's ordinary and usual environment, even when the nursing care takes place in the client's home. Physically, the nursing environment may include elements that are only present in specialized situations that may be different from home, occupational, or recreational settings. Socially, it consists of individuals who are not usually present in the ordinary environment, and it may be lacking the usual social constituents such as family members and friends in the immediate part of the environment. Symbolically, the environment encompasses role expectations that are specific to clients and nurses, subcultural values and ideas, and specialized knowledge systems. Thus, the contents of an environment hold specialized meanings and generate different kinds of influences on a client. Although a nursing environment is a somewhat specialized type of environment, an individual can be viewed to be in the core of an environmental field, moving from one form of specialized environment to another throughout the life cycle. Thus, universal, institutional, and individual forces of nature, combined with human mobility and self-determination, decide in what sorts of specialized forms of environment one gets positioned and for what duration.

Such observations make apparent the difficulty in viewing and analyzing environment in a holistic sense. For this reason, a particularistic approach, taking physical, social, and symbolic environments as separate phenomena, is adopted as an analytic posture in the following sections. While no environment may be conceptualized as having only one of these components completely separately, it appears useful to take different characteristics of environment as the point of departure for theoretical considerations.

## THE MAJOR COMPONENTS OF ENVIRONMENT

### PHYSICAL ENVIRONMENT

Concepts of physical environment are most appropriately found within the domain of a field called human ecology. The main concept in the field of human ecology is *ecosystem*, which is defined as a system of interactions between the various human groups themselves and with the physical and chemical components of the environment. The basic process of an ecosystem is usually considered in terms of energetics, having energy transfer between and among elements of the environment as the basis for changes that evolve. Inherent in this idea of environment is that elements in the environment are capable of generating and exchanging energy and that energy transfer is the elementary form of interaction between elements.

Physical environment has been categorized in various ways. Air, water, and places as used by Hippocrates are persistently used to describe the universalistic world of living. The concept of "place" can be all-encompassing with regard to the constituents that are connected with a spatially and/or geographically defined area. Therefore, a place may mean an urban location of congestion with polluted air, limited open space and vegetation, and crowded with heterogeneous sorts of people.

In general, physical environment is thought to be composed of biotic and abiotic elements. Biotic elements are in various forms, ranging from virus to human beings. Symbiosis as a process has been identified as producing peaceful, mutually advantageous coexistence and growth among many species. A human being as a physical entity in the physical environment takes conceptually a quite different meaning from that of a social being in the social environment. As a physical entity, a person produces and uses heat; occupies space; generates, regenerates, and degenerates its chemical constituents; and has a contiguous surface. Territoriality and crowding are the most commonly studied phenomena in which human beings are taken as physical objects in the environment. Of course, the process by which a person handles the problems of territorial competition and crowding are far more sophisticated than those of other biotic organisms.

Abiotic elements may be distinguished as natural or as artifacts. Although our external world is composed of many and various types of natural physical elements, such as air, water, mountains, rivers, etc., civilization has created and deposited many more abiotic artifactual elements in the environment of modern humanity. We are surrounded by artifacts, starting with clothing as the most proximal ones and extending to satellites orbiting the earth. In addition, we are continuously trying to change the nature and form of the natural physical elements in an attempt to control our surroundings.

Currently, in the field of genetic engineering research, biotic artifacts such as the variant DNA-spliced *E. coli* forms are beginning to be created, arousing suspicions and concerns about contaminating the biosphere with unknown living organisms whose potential effects on humans and the universe are not yet predictable. Genetic engineering poses problems, not only those related to changing the fundamental genetic makeup of organisms, but also associated with the consequences of such manipulations on human existence. Yet, a fascination with control and understanding persists. In a way, the diversity in the available forms of artifacts in modern societies suggests the high level of control humanity has made of its physical environment, and also suggests more possibilities in the future.

Physical environment affects the individual's health in a variety of ways. Nutritional disturbances produced by an undersupply of foodstuffs in different regions of the world are the most obvious. Environmental diseases, such as lead-poisoning, asbestosis, or high altitude headache, as well as infectious diseases, are also well-recognized by-products of the harmful elements in the physical world. In addition, many physical elements of an environment are also responsible for patterning specific life styles, activities, and habits of people, indirectly influencing individuals' statures, physiques, longevity, and health. Furthermore, artifacts produce stimulations such as noise, heat, radiation, and crowding as well as convenience, efficiency, and effectiveness in living conditions. These, in turn, influence an individual's health in both positive and negative ways.

To date, Dubos (1965) has made the most impressive arguments regarding a person's relationships to the environment and his or her capacity to adapt to various environmental elements.

> At a higher level of integration, the organism responds adaptively to many kinds of stimuli by behavior patterns designed to abolish or neutralize the stressor stimuli, or to withdraw from it. Organisms with a highly developed nervous system have several alternative mechanisms of behavioral responses and, furthermore, they possess the ability to ignore some of the stimuli that impinge upon them. The higher the organism is in the evolutionary scale, the more numerous and varied are the types of responses at its disposal and the greater is its ability for selecting limited aspects of the environment to which it responds. The most evolved types of responses are the processes of social adaptation, through which the individual organism and the group modify either their environment or their habits, or both, in order to achieve a way of life better suited to their needs and tastes.[3]

In addition, Dubos postulates that a person's ability to adapt to the environment is influenced by the kinds of symbolic meaning the person attaches to elements in the environment and by the manner with which he or she responds emotionally, that is symbolically, to other human beings. A person's capacity for adaptation is seen as boundless, yet this potentiality can become stifled if a state of adaptedness to environmental conditions is attained and maintained for a prolonged period. A person's adaptive potentiality is stimulated by challenges of unforeseeable threats and changes in the environment, although sudden and profound changes in the environment always pose adaptive difficulties however transitory they may be. In this perspective, Dubos (1965) indicates that health as a state free of pain and disease is a mirage, but when viewed as a state in which environmental challenges are met adaptively for human functioning, it conveys a dynamic meaning.

These ideas suggest that physical environment may be conceptualized in a variety of ways:

1. milieu for functioning,
2. source of stress and stimulation,
3. source for adaptive challenge,
4. symbiotic-interdependent system,
5. spatial construct,
6. object of human control.

In this way, environmental influences on health are thus perceived differently according to the perspectives taken to view the environment. Furthermore, the nursing care environment as a temporary physical environment for a client may be also considered in different terms such as: (a) a milieu for the client's functioning that possesses many restrictive objects; (b) that containing objects and people providing stimulation to the client (e.g., beeping sound of the cardiac monitor); (c) that providing unexpected as well as expected difficulties to the client, such as a new diet; (d) a system of interdependence in which material, energy, and information are exchanged between the elements in the environment and the client; (e) a confinement where there is a limited freedom of movement; or (f) that containing objects for control by the client. Thus, the environmental forces in a nursing care environment are additions to a person's ordinary environment, posing temporary threats to and amenities for a client's life and health.

## SOCIAL ENVIRONMENT

The physical and mental health of an individual depends to a great extent on social factors: the socialization process which he was submitted to by his parents, his present work situation, family life and group affiliation, and the modes of medical treatment he can economically afford and which are culturally prescribed. There is a dynamic relationship between the physical condition of a person and the social structure of which he is a part. Health as a normal condition of the body does not mean the absence of disturbances but rather an effective bodily reaction toward them which continuously reestablishes the precarious equilibrium between different physiological functions.[4]

The basic propositions by which we consider social environment an important factor for human health are that a successful and satisfying social life is partly responsible for health, and that the quality of social life is determined by characteristics of social environment and a person's handling of social environmental forces.

Evidence indicates that the physical and mental health of an individual is closely tied to one's attitudes toward life and living (Vaillant, 1979), one's style of coping (Lazarus, 1976), and the amount of understanding, love, and companionship one receives (Lynch, 1977). In postulating the notion that effective social adjustment is positively related to health and longevity, Wolf states that one prototype of the healthy, long-lived, fulfilled person may be the fine symphony conductor, an individual who is persistently responsive to physical, intellectual, and aesthetic challenges and, also, who is more or less continuously the recipient of approbation from his audiences (1981, p. 11).

More specifically, an individual's health is affected by the quality of social forces: opportunities in, and quality of, social interaction and affiliation; affective quality in dominant social situations, such as family, work, or neighborhood settings; and stresses generated in social life. A person learns how to cope with stresses and develops patterns of behaviors in dealing with life tasks and crises through the socialization process that takes place primarily in family and primary social groups (Kaplan, 1971). In addition, a person also learns to behave according to social expectations, expectations of self and others that may be universal to all situations or particular to a given context. In this view, people having the same "diagnostic" condition may be healthy or sick according to the way they respond within the prescribed, expected, and desired rules of their social contexts of actions and interactions.

Conceptualization of social environment is rooted in the tradition of sociology. As stated earlier, Parsons considers social objects, that is, individuals and collectivities of individuals, as making up significant aspects of the object world in which an individual is engaged in actions and interactions. One crucial distinction between social environment and physical environment is the ability of social objects to act according to will. A person acts upon and reacts in a situation not only to "stimuli" given to him or her, but more importantly according to symbolic interpretations of the stimuli that are made unconsciously and consciously. Thus, social environment represents multiplicity of human characteristics composed of organism-personality complexes.

In a social environment, a person brings with him or her different genetic and developmental characteristics, personality, social capabilities, and personal history. But because a person moves within society, within carefully defined systems of power, prestige, and expectations, the social environment of any given individual at any given time takes on somewhat predictable characteristics. In addition, the structures of society in which we live provide reasons for the coming together of certain individuals in a social situation. Hence, a child of a kibbutz is surrounded by many children and other adults in addition to his or her parents, and these comprise the ordinary social environment. In contrast, a child of an ordinary American family is probably surrounded by one sibling and parents.

The fabrics of social environment not only are reflected by individual characteristics but also by the meanings that are attached to them. To Parsons, individuals in interactions are oriented to such actions in three respects: cathectic, cognitive, and evaluative orientations (1951). This conceptualization can be extended for our exposition to classify conceptual meanings of social objects in an environment—to wit, each individual in a social environment projects to another person certain meanings through his or her presence, actions, or interactions with respect to *affection* (cathexis), *information* (cognition), and *appraisal* (evaluation). In turn, such meanings are translated by the second person as forces having certain values to him or her according to the social rules under which most social acts take place. In this way, social objects and the significance of them to the person become personalized within the boundary of social rules. Thus, recognizing social objects, a person literally embraces those individuals into his or her environment, and accepts affective, informational, and evaluative meanings from them. For example, a girl in a crowd takes in meanings and orientations of a special form when she sees or knows the presence of a close friend among them, which also would be entirely different from the meanings and orientations she takes in when she believes that she is totally among strangers.

Analytically, the social environment can thus be conceptualized in two ways: (a) in qualitative terms as social forces that are determined by characteristics of individuals in the environment generating affective, informational, and evaluative meanings; and (b) in quantitative terms as in social network and boundary, which are related to frequency and extent of affiliation, contact, and influence. As for the first conceptualization, such phenomena as social support, expectation congruency, competition, social control, etc., are but a few aspects of social environment that have been found to have influence on health status and health behaviors. For example, social control that exists in work situations has been found to contribute to the occurrence of coronary health diseases (Garfield, 1979), while Bruhm and Wolf (1979) attributed changes in social integration to increased rate of heart attack. Social support also has been shown to influence the occurrence of mental disorders, to modify illness responses to life's stresses, and to affect the rate and quality of health services utilization (Boswell, 1969; McKinlay, 1972; Cassel, 1976; Cobb, 1976; Gore, 1978; and Cohen and Sokolovsky, 1979).

As for the second conceptualization, marginality, social isolation, and disengagement have been found to have relationships with emotional distress and early death.

Within the social context of nursing practice, it is clear that the environment of health care produces specific meanings and contents to a client who is advertently or inadvertently affected by individuals in the situation. Nurses as social objects are the sources of affection, information, and appraisal to the client. Nurses provide a client with warmth, personal attachment, or emotional neutrality; impart new knowledge about health and health care; and appraise the client's behaviors as appropriate or inappropriate, dispensing approval/ disapproval or rewards/punishments.

Clients, especially in nurse-controlled settings such as hospitals, are vulnerable to nurses' decisions to be an immediate part of their social environments, for clients are potential or sometimes unavoidable social objects of the nurses' environments. Distancing, avoiding, and several forms of social interaction have been found to be used by nurses to control clients' behaviors in hospital settings (Baider, 1976; and Maslach, 1979). In addition, nurses are also frequently in a position to control the makeup of the client's social environment, by limiting visiting hours, allowing rooming-in of family members for hospital care, or by placing the client in hospice care. The social environment of dying patients in our society has been studied and criticized for its impersonality and deception. Such a context seems to prescribe social interactions between professionals, family members, and patients that are psychologically destructive and detrimental to patients (Baider, 1976; and Erickson and Hyerskay, 1975).

Thus, considerations of social environment for human health from the nursing perspective need to be made in two ways: as that influencing the health status of individuals through direct or intervening processes, and as that contributing to the process of health care and nursing practice.

## SYMBOLIC ENVIRONMENT

The meaning of symbolic environment is closely connected with the ''sociality'' of human history and concomitently with social environment. It is not possible to imagine symbolic environment without people or language and historical accumulation of our thoughts, emotions, and acts. Objects of symbolic environment, if we can call them objects, are bound to human histories and human minds. Symbolic environment is composed of *shared ideas on various levels:* cultural values, scientific knowledge, social norms, and role expectations, among others. Analytically, an individual's ideas, attitudes, feelings, and knowledge belong to the individual as inherent parts of the individual, hence such elements become intrinsic parts of the individual as a social object. In contrast, ''shared ideas'' are considered to represent the symbolic environment. In a strict sense, ''shared ideas'' belong to no one and to everyone. Symbolic environment has meaning for human life to the extent that our behaviors and human happenings are modified and patterned by them, and insofar as the person is able to take in the meanings of symbols. Therefore, for instance, an infant of three days old has a very limited symbolic environment, compared to a child of four years old. In addition, the extent of the symbolic environment is irrelevant to the physical proximity of physical and social objects. Hence, the astronauts on the surface of the moon can be presumed to have had as extensive a symbolic environment as when they were on earth.

Sociologists consider such shared ideas functional to societies and social life. Cultural and social values and rules curtail human actions and control the fierce competition and conflict possible among individuals left alone to act according to their personal needs. Symbolic environment allows a client to behave in the ''right'' ways, while it permits a nurse to provide reinforcements for ''right'' behaviors. Symbolic environment provides a common reference point from which individuals in social as well as in solitary circumstances recognize and perform valued actions.

Viewed from the nursing perspective, symbolic environment has three specific components: (a) those elements that define ''what health and illness are,'' and ''what one 'should' do about one's health and illness''; (b) those elements that define available resources in dealing with health issues; and (c) those elements that prescribe role-relationships in health care.

The first component refers to *cultural values and social norms* regarding health and health behaviors. Cultural definitions of mental illness and controversial "deviance" are good examples of how individuals in a given culture interpret such behaviors as depression and homosexuality. Social norms exert pressures on individuals to behave in certain ways, as evidenced in fertility rates in societies, or in health-care seeking behaviors for certain kinds of symptoms. Thus, symbolic environment in the forms of cultural values and social norms exist for individuals exerting influences on their behaviors of many sorts.

Durkheim's study (1951) of societal differences in suicidal rates of nineteenth century Europe provides an important background from which the proposition regarding symbolic environment can be reaffirmed: Ills of societies need to be examined and explained to a great extent by what Durkheim called "collective tendencies," i.e., social conscience. The effects of symbolic environment on an individual's behaviors may be summarized as was done by Durkheim in relation to suicide rates.

> At any given moment the moral constitution of society establishes the contingent of voluntary deaths. There is, therefore, for each people a collective force of a definite amount of energy, impelling men to self-destruction. The victim's acts which at first seem to express only his personal temperament are really the supplement and prolongation of a social condition which they express externally.[5]

Social conscience as a form of symbolic environment provides a context in which members of a society evaluate the quality of life and behavioral consequences—thus, the occurrence of actual illness conditions and labeling of them are influenced by moral forces in societies.

The second component of the symbolic environment encompasses elements of *social institutions,* such as science, education, and polity. Scientific knowledge and technology are the major institutional elements that exist as shared ideas in this sense. Fabrega (1980) contends that both health-care seeking behaviors and health-care providing behaviors are determined by theories of illness that are present and shared in a given society. This component of symbolic environment provides a general frame of reference from which a certain level of expectations for control and recovery from illness is formulated in individuals. In primitive societies, this component was mainly composed of notions about supernatural (demonic or godly) influences on human existence. In addition, this component encompasses those symbolic aspects of a society that are defined by structures of institutions such as political, economic, labor, and health-care systems. Renaud (1975) argues that capitalist societies are constrained in their problem-solving endeavor relative to health by their economic structure. Health-care providing behaviors appear to be different according to institutionalized structures of health care in different societies.[6]

The third component is more closely tied to social situations and refers to *rules of behaviors for social roles.* Individuals who come together in a social situation assume certain social roles that are congruent with the situation, and behave in accordance with mutual expectations and rules that have been socially learned. Parsons (1951) describes the sick-role expectations in modern Western societies as: (a) the person recognizing his or her state of illness considers this state undesirable and wants to get better, (b) the person is not considered to be responsible for his or her condition, (c) the person is excused from ordinary social role obligations, and (d) the person seeks professional help and cooperates with the health-care givers. The role expectations of helper and helpee are also socially derived and usually known to client and practitioner who come together in service settings. Because such expectations do not belong to persons, although they are held by them and internalized by them, such elements are parts of the symbolic environment.

Important questions regarding the symbolic environment from the nursing perspective should deal with the nature of shared ideas, the extent to which such shared ideas govern behaviors, and characteristics of sharing among individuals in a given society with respect to health, health behavior, and nurse-client relations. When a society goes through disintegration, or when a persisting conflict exists among individuals having different vested interests, one might experience a lack of consensus in behavioral expectations, thus creating chaotic actions. In such cases, the symbolic environment is not enhancing to individuals' behaviors.

## SELECTED CONCEPTUAL ANALYSES

Among many possible concepts within the domain of environment appropriate for studying from the nursing perspective, *sensory deprivation, social support,* and *sick-role expectation* have been selected for analysis in this section. These were selected from the examples listed in Table 7. Table 7 presents examples of concepts in the domain of environment that are thought to be appropriate for theoretical considerations from the nursing perspective. Sensory deprivation is considered as an example of physical environment phenomena; social support as that of social environment phenomena; and sick-role expectation as an example of symbolic environment phenomena. The main purpose of this section is to show how a first-level analytical approach is used to gain conceptual and empirical understanding of phenomena within the domain of environment. Each concept is analyzed with respect to (a) definitional clarification and conceptual meanings as reflected in the literature, (b) measurement and operationalization of concepts as a step toward an empirical analysis, and (c) the concept's relationships with other concepts that are important in nursing. The strategy and rationale for the conceptual analysis were discussed in detail in Chapter 2, and that rationale is adopted in this section for the analyses of sensory deprivation, social support, and sick-role expectation.

**TABLE 7. Examples of Concepts in the Domain of Environment for Study in the Nursing Perspective**

| Environmental Component | Concept |
|---|---|
| Physical environment | Space, territory, proxemics |
| | Time |
| | Ecosystem |
| | Energy |
| | Noise |
| | Crowding |
| | Sensory deprivation |
| | Sensory overload |
| | Pathogen |
| | Heat |
| Social environment | Social support |
| | Competition |
| | Social control |
| | Social isolation |
| | Disengagement |
| | Affective milieu |
| | Marginality |
| | Proximity |
| Symbolic environment | Power structure (authority) |
| | Role-expectation |
| | Sick-role |
| | Expertise |
| | Value |
| | Norm |
| | Morality |
| | Knowledge |
| | Rationality |
| | Positivism |

## SENSORY DEPRIVATION

**Definition**

Environment is the source of sensory inputs for human perceptions: sound, color, form, texture, temperature, and many other physical characteristics are perceived and sensed in order for a person to make assessments about the world around him or her and gauge his or her position in relation to them. A person recognizes familiar objects and persons, learns about new objects, and guards against unfamiliar objects that are judged to be potentially threatening. A person's life in a vacuum, if that is at all possible, may represent an ultimate state of absence of sensory input to the person. Persons placed in solitary confinements in jails or hospitals have been found to create sensory inputs by banging their heads on walls, scratching, or screaming. Lack of sensory input is threatening to adults who have learned to perceive the world through the senses. Thus, it tends to create a sense of disconnectedness with the world in persons when they are placed in a sensory-deprived environment. People receiving no sensory input may begin to doubt their own existence. Infants who are placed in deprived (sensory) environment have also been found to assume the condition of "deprivation dwarfism" (Gardner, 1976).

The basic premises for the occurrence of such phenomena are that the human brain matures and develops through sensory stimulation, and that human behavior is shaped by functional and structural organization of information that occurs in the brain. Hebb's attempt (1947) to explain perceptual behavior in relation to the function of the central nervous system was the first link made between behavior and sensory experience. He postulated that perceptual behavior is influenced by early experience with deprivation of vision and other sense modalities and that monotonous, unchanging stimulation resulted in a disorganization of the ability and capacity to think.

By definition, then, sensory deprivation is a lack or reduction of sensory stimulation in several different forms, varying in terms of intensity, duration, and characteristics. As early as 1949, Bakan described sensory deprivation as a state in which an organism is deprived of normal, complex sensory stimulation from the external environment for a specified period (Brownfield, 1972). Yet, there has been little agreement in the use and definition of the term describing the phenomenon. Rossi (1969) cites 25 different terms used more or less interchangeably with sensory deprivation in the literature. The problem of definition has been complicated because of the nature of research being done in the field. Many research studies adopt experimental conditions to "induce" the phenomenon of sensory deprivation artificially, and such procedural terms have been used interchangeably to denote the phenomenon in a limited sense.

In general, there are two broadly and distinctly different conceptualizations of sensory deprivation: (a) a state in which the focus is the environment and (b) a state in which the focus is the individual organism experiencing the deprivation. The first conceptualization considers the phenomenon strictly in terms of the environmental characteristics as a lack, reduction, or monotonicity of sensory stimulation present in the environment. On the other hand, the second conceptualization refers either to the condition of the person being in a "deprived" state, or to a process in which a phenomenological experience of deprivation takes place in the person (Rossi, 1969). It appears that there is an analytical value in considering the phenomenon in such two separate ways. Our interest in the conceptualization of sensory deprivation is in line with the first type in which the environmental characteristics are the major focus.

Suedfeld (1969) categorizes sensory deprivation in terms of three major characteristics: the reduction of stimulus-input levels, the reduction of stimulus-variability, and sensory-social isolation and confinement. Although these three characteristics have somewhat distinct meanings, there is a circularity in meaning-relationships among them. Invariably, in nonexperimental situations, a reduction of stimulus-variability that is produced by monotonous stimulation will result in a reduction of stimulus-input levels, and vice versa. In addition, sensory-social isolation and confinement frequently accompany both a reduction of stimulus-variability and a reduction of stimulus-input levels.

### Differentiation of the Concept from Isolation
The phenomenon of isolation encompasses a broader conceptual meaning than that of sensory deprivation. Isolation suggests removing a person to a confined area without allowing normal contacts with the external world. Brownfield (1972) suggests four kinds of isolation: (a) confinement in which a person is placed in a limited space, restraining the freedom of movement and in which sensory deprivation may vary according to the nature of the space; (b) separation in which a person is placed in an environment where personal contacts with particular persons, places, or things are not allowed, and which brings about deprivation of special kinds of sensory inputs; (c) removal from the total environment in which a person is placed in an environment of reduced normal stimulation or no stimulation, such as solitary confinement; and (d) monotony of stimulation in which a person is exposed to unchanging, invariable, and boring sensory inputs that eventually lose their ability to elicit responses.

Thus, the phenomenon of isolation may be induced by unconscious or conscious acts by a person (i.e., psychologically based), such as voluntary deprivation, self-punishment, or social isolation because of fear, religious beliefs, or conscience, and also may be imposed by external forces such as immobility, old age, loss of sensory ability, or impoverished early experience.

In general, isolation encompasses the aspects of social and psychological separation, while sensory deprivation is associated with the characteristics of the environment in terms of its sensory stimulation. Of course, isolation is a situation in which sensory deprivation is likely to occur.

In differentiating the phenomenon of isolation and sensory deprivation, one source of confusion has been in the use of experimental "isolation" techniques in sensory deprivation research. Such techniques invariably combine reduction and monotonization of stimulation in isolating experimental subjects in order to manipulate sensory inputs.

### Operationalization
Sensory deprivation has been operationalized in research in two specific ways: as an environment in which there is a reduction of intensity of sensory inputs, and as an environment in which there is homogeneous and unpatterned input. Both

of these operational definitions have been used to create an experimental environment.

The first type of operationalization generally refers to an experimental condition deliberately lacking in sensory stimulation, such as silence and darkness as used by Myers and his colleagues (1963). The second type of operationalization refers to an experimental environment in which there is a limitation in the variability of sensory input such as constant masking of sensory input or white noise and diffused light, as used in McGill studies (Scott, Bexton, Heron, and Downe, 1959).

Operationalizations used in such experimental conditions create conceptual complications in that, when an environment has been manipulated to reduce sensory input, the remaining sensory elements in the environment take on different perceptual meanings to the person exposed to such an environment.

In addition, in most research studies, sensory deprivation has been operationalized to include the aspects of visual and auditory stimuli, with little emphasis on tactile, olfactory, kinesthetic, gustatory, and proprioceptive sense modalities. However, sensory deprivation operationalized in developmental research, in many cases, includes the concept of multisensory deprivation. Deprivation of visual, auditory, tactile, and movement stimulations has been used specifically to indicate the deprivation of novelty in stimulation in those developmental studies. Stimulation for new learning is absent as a result of such deprivation (Reisen and Zilbert, 1975).

Operationalization of sensory deprivation referring to naturally occurring environmental conditions has been limited to hospital and nursing-home settings (Worrell, 1971). The most commonly studied settings of sensory deprivation in the health-care situation are: private room for a coronary patient; private room for a surgical patient, especially a patient with cardiac surgery; elderly patient, especially the elderly who has decreased sensory abilities such as blindness, hearing loss, or other perceptual loss; "isolation" or "seclusion" room; hospital settings for immobilized patients such as those with stroke, in traction, or with spinal cord injury; and private room for a patient with eye surgery. These kinds of nursing care situations have a reduced rather than a complete lack of sensory stimulation and usually provide monotonous or unchanging stimulations of sounds and visual objects. Monotonous sensory input of a mute nature has been defined as perceptual deprivation, differentiating it from the general concept of sensory deprivation.

Perceptual deprivation, defined as such, is more commonly detectable in clinical, practice settings. Newman (1981) studied the isolette environment of preterm infants, in which the isolette environment is perceived as an auditory environment of high ground noise and intrusive sound of a disturbing nature. This isolette environment is conceived to provide infants with a situation in which human sounds are filtered by such ground noises. It is thus seen as producing perceptual deprivation in infants.

Social isolation, confinement, withdrawal, and neglect have also been used to denote sensory deprivation in sociological and psychological studies. In particular, the isolation and confinement of the elderly in single-occupancy hotel rooms in which variation in sensory input is lacking for an extended period of time have been considered as an environment of sensory deprivation for the elderly.

It appears that operationalization of sensory deprivation depends on one's definition of the term and can vary from deprivation of one sensory modality to a complete deprivation of sensory input as well as monotony of sensory input.

## Relationship with Other Concepts

Most of the studies in the field of sensory deprivation may be categorized into those relating sensory deprivation to the developmental consequences and those relating sensory deprivation to other behavioral aberrations such as hallucination.

There are many studies in the first category, emphasizing the maturational effects on specific senses and the general behavioral and developmental consequences. Animal and human studies found relationships between early visual experience (or the lack of it) and visual preference, indicating the influence of early sensory stimulation on sensory maturation (Tees, Midgley, and Bruinsma, 1980; and Annis and Frost, 1973). In addition, Prescott (1980) suggests that sensory deprivation during early development leads to stimulus-seeking behaviors relative to the deprived sensory systems, and further that somatosensory, affectional deprivation from isolation rearing may be responsible for violent behaviors toward self and others. Alcoholism and drug abuse as stimulus-seeking behaviors have been postulated to be the results of such deprivation. Thus, the individual is assumed to be attempting to gain the sensory stimulation that was deprived early in life.

Deprivation dwarfism has also been suggested as a secondary effect of hypopituitarism produced by sensory deprivation in animals and humans (Patton and Gardner, 1975; Powell, Brasel, and Blizzard, 1967; Wolff and Money, 1973; and Brown, 1976).

One of the major variables identified as a consequence of sensory deprivation in the second category of studies is hallucinatory activity such as visual imagery and test performance found in McGill studies (Bexton, Heron, and Scott, 1954). Zuckerman (1969) explains the phenomenon of hallucination as a self-aroused imagery perceived by a person because of a lack of competing sensory inputs. A person in an environment without patterned and changing stimulation eventually may become sensitized to more organized images whose site of origin lies higher in the nervous system and that may be intensified by a high state of arousal or by reduction in competing stimuli, thus appearing as visual imageries localized in space in front of the person.

It also has been shown that visual deprivation is associated with an increased tactual acuity, pain sensitivity, auditory discrimination, and olfactory and gustatory sensitivity. In addition, other single-modality deprivation can also produce behavioral changes (Zubek, 1969). Biochemical changes, especially that of steroids and endorphins, have been the concerns of many current studies, suggesting a linkage between sensory deprivation and behavioral changes mediated by internal processes of biochemical synthesis (Zubek, 1969; and Prescott, 1980).

Zuckerman (1969) and Suedfeld (1969) have examined various theoretical approaches used in studies of sensory deprivation and found diversity in the explanations and in inclusion of various types of dependent variables in explanations.

In the nursing literature, sensory deprivation has been handled in a casual, cursory manner. Theoretical or empirical writings are rarely found on this subject, although sensory deprivation in practice settings is often seen in hospitalized and nursing-home patients, and its deleterious effect on patients has been observed by nurses. Complaints of hallucination and confusion by postsurgical patients, elderly patients, and immobilized patients have been reported by many nurses in clinical case studies and at clinical conferences. The importance of sensory deprivation for a nursing study is apparent, in view of the fact that most of the naturally occurring sensory deprivations are present in health-care environments, and also that effects of sensory deprivation are general and nonspecific to the person and his or her development. Furthermore, sensory deprivation as a phenomenon of the client's environment may complicate the client's recovery from illness in a rather complex manner. The environment of nursing care may inadvertently be the source of sensory deprivation to the client, thus becoming a deleterious rather than enhancing surrounding for health-recovery and health-maintenance.


## SOCIAL SUPPORT

### Definition
In general, social support refers to positive, reinforcing attitudes generated by individuals in social relations to each other. Although it is this "supportiveness" that is central to the concept, it has been used in research synonymously with social network, social bond, and social integration. This has created some confusion in the theoretical formulation of the concept.

The main source of such confusion is embedded in viewing the source of "support," i.e., social relation and social network, interchangeably with the nature of "support." For example, Antonovsky (1979) states that social support is the extent to which a person is lodged in social networks to which the person is committed; and Myers et al. (1975), Eaton (1978), and Brown et al. (1975) also conceptualize social support in terms of the extensiveness of social relationships. In addition, "meaningful social contact" (Cassel, 1976), availability of confidants (Miller and Ingham, 1976), human companionship (Lynch, 1977), social bond (Henderson, 1977 and 1980), and social network (cf. Mueller, 1980; and Norbeck, 1981) have been used to make inferences about social support. Although the assumption is that social relationships and networks provide support, evidence indicates that the relationship between the intensity, size, and extensity of a social network and social support is not linear.[7]

Cobb (1976) and Turner (1980) consider social support in terms of information. Social support is viewed on the basis of three types of information:

1. Affective information—information suggestive of being loved and cared for.
2. Information of worthiness—information suggestive of being valued and esteemed.
3. Information of partisanship—information suggestive of belonging to mutually influencing social relations.

In a similar fashion, Kaplan and his colleagues (1977) define social support as the degree to which an individual's needs for affection, security, approval, belongingness, and identity are "met" through social interaction. This definition also assumes that the person's perception is an integral part of social support.

What does not emerge from these definitions is the suggestion of different kinds of support that are possible in social relations. This question can be raised by linking the conceptualization of social network as the source of social support and the reference-group theory proposed by Merton (1968). The reference-group theory suggests that individuals use their social contacts as the framework for receiving reinforcements, support, and evaluations when making behavioral choices and in expressing ideas and attitudes. Hence, the information one receives from relationships with others may be both emotional (affective) and cognitive (evaluative), and both types of information may be "supportive" to the person in general or in specific situations. Therefore, it is possible to conceptualize social support as information generated to a person in social relations, information that has either general affective or specific instrumental meaning of support.

## Operationalization

Different definitions of social support used in the field have resulted in varied and sometimes limiting operationalizations of the concept. In defining social support in terms of more "affective" than "instrumental" information, Turner (1980) used self-evaluation of the perceived level of information generated by others to indicate the level of social support. He used vignettes developed by Kaplan (1977) as the basis of self-evaluation. LaRocco, House, and French (1980) also operationalized social support as perceived psychological and tangible support from supervisors, co-workers, spouse, family, and friends. They specifically defined social support as "emotional supportiveness." A limitation in this kind of operationalization is the lack of objective criteria to attest to the fit between perceived information and actual supportiveness present in social relations.

It is problematic to assume that "perceived" support equals "real" support present in the social environment. This difficulty is based on two issues: (a) perception can be influenced by a person's interpretation of meanings attached to self, others, situation, and happenings; and (b) supportiveness may not be apparent until actual "incidents" or occasions call for mobilization of support being offered or already given by others. The first problem points up the need for objective criteria for interpretations, and the second issue raises a further question regarding the need for differentiating generalized versus contextual or specialized support.

A more inclusive operationalization of the concept of social support is found in several studies. Gore (1978) operationalizes social support on three dimensions: (a) a person's perception of supportiveness of significant others; (b) frequency of activity outside the home with significant others that indicates amount of social interaction; and (c) perceived opportunity for engaging in supportive and satisfying social activities. Similarly, Lin and colleagues (1979) define social support as support accessible to an individual through social ties to other individuals, groups, and the larger community. They measure the concept in terms of the degree of social interaction and involvement and the level of social adjustment. Other researchers also have operationalized social support on multidimensional levels, including social relations, perceptions, and type of support.[8]

However, operationalization of social support is in need of consensus. While most researchers consider the sources of support in terms of significant others, few research studies have included support from the community at large and from lay-support systems as important components of the total social support system. Furthermore, operational difficulties in differentiating the nature of affective and instrumental support and in attaining consensus regarding perceived support vis-a-vis "apparent" support need to be addressed.

## Relationships with Other Concepts
Social support has been used to explain various phenomena in an individual's life. The basic notion is that an individual's behaviors may be explained by factors in his or her social environment such as social network, interaction patterns, or structures of social institutions. This notion extends the explanation of human behavior beyond the attributes of individuals themselves. Social support

has been applied in many studies to explain the relationships among social environment, occurrence and management of stress, health status, and other social behaviors. Social support has been viewed to have mediating or buffering effects on the way individuals handle stress, modify illness responses associated with life's stresses, and affect the rate and quality of health-services utilization.

In her study of the effects of social support in moderating the health consequences of unemployment, Gore (1978) suggested that the loss of self-worthiness through unemployment and confounded by the lack of social support contributed to negative health consequences. Myers et al. (1975) also concluded that persons with high social integration scores seem better able to cope with the impact of life's stresses, alluding to the idea that the accessibility to social support and integration contribute to better coping with stress. The same mechanism has also been proposed by many other researchers.[9]

Evidence suggesting the relationships between the use of health services and social support are confusing. Salloway and Dillon (1973) found that different types of networks influenced the degree of speed with which one used health services. Large friend-networks may also be influential in encouraging a person to seek medical care. On the other hand, health-care seeking behaviors may be more influenced by the kinds of advice one receives rather than by the sources of the support.

Effects of social support on a client's compliance to health-care practices and therapies have also been frequently documented in the nursing literature. It appears that clients who have support in their daily life are more likely to adhere to many unfavored and/or unpleasant regimens, compared to those individuals who are lacking in social reinforcement.

From the nursing perpective, three major phenomena seem important for study in relation to social support:

1. the individual's patterns of coping with stress;
2. the individual's reactions and behaviors related to illness experiences;
3. the individual's compliance behaviors with regard to health-care regimens.


## SICK-ROLE EXPECTATION

### Definition
Parsons (1951) defines illness as a state of disturbance in the "normal" functioning of the total human individual, including both the state of the organism as a biological being, and the state of his or her personal and social adjustments. It is therefore viewed as a form of "social" deviance that requires management by mechanisms of social control. Hence, the sick role as "the institutionalized

expectation system" is conceptualized by Parsons as the mechanism of social control for an individual's illness.

Parsons (1951) proposed that the institutionalized expectation system of the sick role is composed of four aspects:

1. A sick person expects an exemption from normal social role respon-sibilities, an exemption of varying extent according to the nature and severity of the illness, and expects the exemption to be legiti-matized by someone and to members of immediate social groups.
2. A sick person is relieved of "being responsible" for his or her ill-ness.
3. A sick person is expected to want to get well, since the state of be-ing ill is viewed as undesirable.
4. A sick person is expected and is compelled to submit to technically competent help.

Twaddle (1979) suggests that the conceptualization of the sick role is spe-cifically tied to the view that "sickness" is a social label for the state of being unwell, or "nonhealth." He also differentiates three states that comprise "non-health": *disease,* referring to biological capacities; *illness,* encompassing subjec-tive or psychological meanings; and *sickness,* referring to a social aspect. Thus, to be sick is to have certain rights and obligations ascribed by social role-expecta-tions, while to be diseased means to have signs and symptoms of disturbance, and to be ill is to feel deviated from well feelings.

Much of the debate regarding the concept of the sick role has centered around the four components identified by Parsons as the universal construct of the sick role. Freidson (1970), especially, argues that the expectation of the ex-emption from social role obligations may be limited to certain types of disease; that societies attribute the causes of some illnesses to sick persons themselves; that the expectation to seek and cooperate with professional help can be univer-sal neither for all types of illness nor for all societies; and that the basic constructs of Parsons are rooted in the value structures and institutional development of Western, modernized societies, and are thus not applicable to nonwestern soci-eties.

Parsons proposed the sick role as containing symbolic properties of a soci-ety, especially those of American society. This role is an institutionalized basis of social control for illness in a society. Contents of the sick role reflect the major value structures of a given society. Therefore, it may be more useful to define the sick role as a system of expectations that are institutionalized and accepted as the general "guidelines" for defining the meanings of sickness and for model be-haviors of the person who is sick. This goes along with Twaddle's notion that the sick role is an effect variable to be explained on a global scale with respect to soci-etal differences (1979). The sick role, then, is a system of general norms and expectations that provide a context for "rightful" behaviors for sick individuals in a given society or culture.

## Operationalization

The operational definition of the sick role has suffered from the confusion that occurred when researchers applied the concept in research. Many researchers included both "expectations" and "behaviors" to indicate the sick role. For example, Twaddle (1969) included both stated expectations for behaviors and the actual behaviors to indicate the sick-role formulation, confounding the role-expectations that are tied to the role-behaviors.

Probably Gordon's study of a large population sample of New York City (1966) is the only one that operationalized the sick-role concept as the generally held expectations for persons who are sick. As a system of value consensus and expectations for role behaviors, the concept needs to be operationalized on a general level, that is, at a societal level or for subsectors of a given society. For it to have any conceptual meaning as a concept representing phenomena in the symbolic environment, it is necessary to operationalize it in terms of "generally" held expectations, i.e., consensus, rather than as an individual's convictions.

## Relationships with Other Concepts

There are three distinct theoretical and empirical questions related to the sick-role concept that appear to be relevant to the nursing perspective.[10]

1. What are the contents of the sick role, and what are the variations of such contents?
2. In what ways are variations explained? What are the relationships between the sick-role expectations and the individual's sickness behaviors?
3. To what extent does the "sharedness" of the sick-role expectations between the professionals and the clients influence health-care behaviors?

The first question is concerned with the descriptive validation of the sick role and focuses on the nature of institutionalization of role expectations. As indicated earlier, very little work has been done to examine the universality of the four aspects of the sick role formulated by Parsons. Segall (1972) explored the sick-role expectations held by hospitalized female patients, and found that only (a) the dimension of undesirability of illness and (b) the expectation for striving to get well were agreed upon as sick-role expectations held in common by patients. This questions the validity of the four dimensions as the universally held expectations of the sick role.

Several researchers also suggested that the four dimensions of the sick role do not apply to all types of illness. For example, Kosa and Robertson (1969) suggest that the sick role only applies to chronic illness. In contrast, Freidson (1962) argues that the sick role is most appropriate in considering nontrivial, acute illnesses. Furthermore, the legitimacy and social definition of certain illnesses, such as mental illness, alcoholism, or drug addiction, confound the sick role concept whenever a society holds the individual personally responsible for the illness and its consequences. It is also apparent that the prevailing philosophy and knowledge that exist in a given society regarding health, disease, and health-care practices influence the way a system of value expectations becomes institutionalized in a society.

Additionally, since in an earlier section of this chapter it was proposed that the symbolic environment may be considered in terms of proximity to individuals, it is necessary to question whether or not the sick-role expectations are different on a subcultural level or in social stratification sectors. Although some variations in sick-role expectations are found among different socioeconomic status groups (Gordon, 1966; Twaddle, 1969; and Berkanovic, 1972), the question raised by Segall (1976) is still appropriate: Are the dimensions and contents of the sick role similar among people from different segments of society or different population groups?

The second question poses relationships between the sick role as independent variable and individuals' behaviors as dependent variables. The basic assumption stems from Parsons' formulation of the theory of action in which individuals' actions are explained in terms of the actors' motivations, values, and orientations to the situations. Thus, individuals are expected to behave in ways that are in agreement with sick-role expectations. However, evidence indicates that the relationship between sick-role expectations and actual behaviors reflecting such expectations seem modified by many factors. The nature of the illness appears to have a highly modifying effect on whether or not the sick person will assume the sick-role behaviors. A person's other role obligations specified by what Merton calls "role-set" (1968) also seem to influence the behaviors related to assuming the sick role. A person's position in the social stratification system may also determine the presence or absence of opportunities for behaving in accordance with sick-role expectations (Twaddle, 1979).

Furthermore, the degree to which an individual adheres to social norms and identifies with the value structure of society, that is, the degree of social "belongingness" or the level of social assimilation, may influence the way one behaves when sick. This may result from either the presence or the lack of validation and reinforcement offered to individuals who are behaving in a certain fashion. This would be more apparent in cases of socially stigmatized illnesses or of ambiguously defined illnesses such as depression, anorexia nervosa, or essential hypertension.

The question of alignment in sick-role expectations and behaviors between professionals and clients has direct implications for nursing. Nurses' behaviors as well as their beliefs about the sick role certainly influence the approaches nurses use toward clients. Since an assumption of the sick role requires validation of the role by others, especially by the professional, this process of validation requires empirical attention. Wolinsky and Wolinsky (1981) found that physicians do not necessarily legitimatize the sick role for everyone who assumes this role. Legitimation is offered more often to those clients who come from a lower socio-economic background, who are seeking validation from a regular source of professional contact, and who have more frequent contact with medical care. There may be two distinct mechanisms that influence the process of validation and alignment of evaluations: (a) The systems of the sick-role expectations are, in fact, different according to the nature of illness, to the extent that professionals and laypeople define illness differently; and (b) the systems of sick-role expectations vary greatly according to substrata and segments of society, to the extent that a majority of the professionals belong to a specific subculture or substrata that is quite different from that of the general population. Consequences to the clients of disparity and disalignment in the validation of the sick role have not been adequately studied in the field.

It is possible to imagine a case in which a person who considers himself to be sick is turned away by a physician or a nurse. The person may be thought of as a malingerer or not being "ill enough." As a consequence, the person may experience frustration, stress, distrust, or relief in an immediate sense, and the person furthermore learns a new normative basis for symptom evaluation that may influence his or her future behaviors.

As pointed out by Twaddle (1979), conversion of sick-role expectations into behaviors on an individual level hinges on "decisions" made by the person to classify himself or herself as sick. Since all two-category decisions of this kind, e.g., sick versus not sick, or hungry versus not hungry, require a criterion of threshold, the problem rests critically on the decision rules used by individuals. Thus, as the primary validators of the sick role, nurses are frequently exposed to situations of disparity. Or, as participants in the provision of health-care, nurses are in situations where legitimation has already occurred that may or may not align with the nurses' own validation rules. Conflicts of this type may result in negative behaviors toward clients.

## SUMMARY

The purpose of this chapter has been to offer conceptualization of environment as a separate entity from that of client. This is done to sharpen the distinction between phenomena within the domain of client and those phenomena within the domain of environment. Consideration of environmental phenomena in a separate context should also highlight the integration between humanity and the environment. The basic premise for this chapter is the notion that environment is the source of forces exerting influences on a person and his or her existence, and that it is also a context in which living (many facets of it) takes place. Therefore, environment, either taken as a whole or as having many distinct classes of phenomena, is an essential component for theoretical thinking in nursing.

While environment as a unity is considered to have specific meanings when taken as a whole, it is also proposed in this exposition that there are scientific benefits in considering the domain of environment as composed of separate components.

The typology of environment used here includes three qualitative components of a physical, social, and symbolic nature, combined with the two dimensions of space and time. Variability of environment can thus be considered in these terms. The most elementary proposition regarding space might be that the more immediate environmental elements are likely to produce a greater impact on a person than the more remote environmental forces. This proposition of proximity requires both theoretical and empirical examinations, first in a holistic sense, then on a compartmentalized level. Specification of dependent phenomena, i.e., aspects of a person on which the impact of the environment is inferred, depends on the scientific perspective of the study. Hence, from the nursing perspective, we would be mostly interested in explaining certain aspects of health-related states and health-related behaviors as affected by environment.

Time dimension in relation to environment poses two types of variability. Duration of environmental presence is the first variability. Some environmental elements are with us continuously, intermittently, or only fleetingly. Rhythmicity of the presence of environmental elements (that is, regularly appearing or randomly present) is the second variability. In many ways, the temporal aspects of one's environment are closely related to the person's habits and patterns of behavior. Continuous exposure to polluted air has a great impact on the human respiratory system, and at the same time an exposure to a highly potent radioactive substance for a fleeting moment can be fatal.

The aspect of quality is inherent in three components of environment, since these components are thought to be characteristically different. Sensory deprivation, social support, and the sick role as differently conceived characteristics of environment have been considered as independent variables impinging on various dependent phenomena in the domain of client. Biological and chemical aspects of environment have been linked to many disease conditions, ranging from smallpox to cancer. Relationships between health and social and symbolic elements of environment are beginning to be explored. Rheumatoid arthritis, coronary heart disease, hypertension, as well as many psychological stress syndromes and mental illnesses have been linked to unfavorable aspects of environment.

In addition, a person's behaviors in seeking health care, responding to diseases, forming habits of everyday life, as well as gaining patterns of growth and development, and learning and unlearning behaviors and knowledge, also have been found to be related to environmental phenomena of various kinds.

Another important consideration of environment within the nursing frame of reference concerns the environment in which nursing care takes place. The environment of nursing care raises quite different kinds of theoretical and empirical questions for nursing scientists. Elements of such an environment, i.e., physical, social, and symbolic environments, affect not only clients who are placed in it but also the ways in which nursing care is provided. Nurses' actions are to some extent created, developed, modified, and constrained within the given environmental contexts. Studying phenomena of the environment from the nursing perspective, then, requires focusing on relationships between nursing-care variations and environment as well as those between a person's health and health-related behaviors and environment.

## BIBLIOGRAPHY

Ahmed, PI, and Coelho, GV. *Toward a New Definition of Health: Psychosocial Dimensions.* New York: Plenum Press, 1979

Altman, I, and Wohlwill, JF (eds.). *Human Behavior and Environment: Advances in Theory and Research.* New York: Plenum Press, 1976

Altman, I, and Wohlwill, JF (eds.). *Human Behavior and Environment: Environment and Culture,* Vol. 4. New York: Plenum Press, 1980

Andrews GC, Tennant, D, Hewson, D, and Vaillant, G. Life Events, Stress, Social Support, Coping Style, and Risk of Psychological Impairment. *J Nerv Ment Dis* 166: 307–316, 1978

Annis, RC, and Frost, B. Human Visual Ecology and Orientation Anisotropics in Acuity. *Science* 182: 729–731, 1973

Antonovsky, A. Social Class and Illness: A Reconsideration. *Sociol Inquiry* 37: 311–322, 1967

Antonovsky, A. *Health, Stress, and Coping.* San Francisco: Jossey-Bass, 1979

Baider, L. Private Experience and Public Expectation on the Cancer Ward. *Omega* 6: 373–381, 1976

Barker, RG (ed.). *Habitats, Environment, and Human Behavior: Studies in Ecological Psychology and Eco-Behavioral Sciences from Midwest Psychological Field Station, 1947-1972.* San Francisco: Jossey-Bass, 1978

Berkanovic, E. Lay Conceptions of the Sick Role. *Social Forces* 51: 53–64, 1972

Bexton, WH, Heron, W, and Scott, TH. Effects of Decreased Variation in the Sensory Environment. *Can J Psychol* 8: 70–76, 1954

Boughey, AS. *Man and the Environment: An Introduction to Human Ecology and Evolution.* New York: Macmillan, 1971

Brickman, HR. Mental Health and Social Change: An Ecological Perspective. In HP

Dreitzel (ed.): *The Social Organization of Health.* New York: The Macmillan, 1971, pp 15–26

Brown, GM. Endocrine Aspects of Psychosocial Dwarfism. In EJ Sachar (ed.): *Hormones, Behavior, and Psychopathology.* New York: Raven Press, 1976

Brown GW, Bhrolchaim, MN, and Harris, T. Social Class and Psychiatric Disturbances Among Women in an Urban Population. *Sociology* 9: 225–254, 1975

Brownfield, CA. *The Brain Benders: A Study of the Effects of Isolation,* Second enlarged edition. New York: Exposition Press, 1972

Bruhn, JG, and Wolf, S. *The Roseto Story: An Anatomy of Health.* Norman, Oklahoma: University of Oklahoma Press, 1979

Cassel, J. Psychosocial Processes and "Stress": Theoretical Formulations. *Int J Health Serv* 4: 471–482, 1974

Cassel, J. The Contribution of the Social Environment to Host Resistance. *Am J Epidemiol* 104: 107–122, 1976

Cobb, S. Social Support as a Moderator of Life Stress. *Psychosom Med* 38: 300–314, 1976

Cobb, S, and Kasl, SV. *Termination: The Consequences of Job Loss.* Cincinnati, Ohio: DHEW (NIOSH) Publication No. 77–224, 1977

Cohen, CI, and Sokolovsky, J. Health-Seeking Behavior and Social Network of the Aged Living in Single-Room Occupancy Hotels. *J Am Geriatr Soc* 27: 270–278, 1979

Dean, A, and Lin, N. The Stress-Buffering Role of Social Support. *J Nerv Ment Dis* 165: 403–417, 1977

Dobzhansky, T. *The Biology of Ultimate Concern.* New York: The New American Library, 1967

Dohrenwend, BS, and Dohrenwend, BP. *Stressful Life Events: Their Nature and Effects.* New York: John Wiley, 1974

Dreitzel, HP. Introduction: The Social Organization of Health. In HP Dreitzel (ed.): *The Social Organization of Health.* New York: Macmillan, 1971, pp vi–xvii

Dubos, R. *Man Adapting.* New Haven: Yale University Press, 1965

Dubos, R. *So Human an Animal.* New York: Charles Scribner's Sons, 1968

Dubos, R. *Man, Medicine, and Environment.* New York: Frederick A. Praeger, 1968

Durkheim, E. *Suicide: A Study in Sociology,* Trans. by JA Spaulding and G Simpson. New York: The Free Press, 1951

Eaton, WW. Life Events, Social Supports, and Psychiatric Symptoms: A Reanalysis of the New Haven Data. *J Health Soc Behav* 19: 230–234, 1978

Einstein, A. *Relativity: The Special and General Theory.* New York: Crown, 1961

Erickson, RC, and Hyerskay, BJ. The Dying Patient and the Double-bind Hypothesis. *Omega* 5: 287–298, 1975

Fabrega, H, Jr. *Disease and Social Behavior: An Interdisciplinary Perspective.* Cambridge: MIT Press, 1974

Fabrega, H, Jr. The Scientific Usefulness of the Idea of Illness. *Perspect Biol Med* 22: 545, 1979

Feibleman, JK. The Artificial Environment. In J Lenihan and W Fletcher (eds.): *The*

*Built Environment: Environment and Man,* Vol. 8. New York: Academic Press, 1978, pp 145–168

Fox, RC. *Essays in Medical Sociology.* New York: John Wiley, 1979

Freedman, DG. *Human Sociobiology: A Holistic Approach.* New York: The Free Press, 1979

Freidson, E. Medical Sociology. *Current Sociology* 10/11, 1962

Freidson, E. *Profession of Medicine.* New York: Dodd, Mead, 1970a

Freidson, E. *Professional Dominance.* New York: Atherton Press, 1970b

Gardner, LI. Deprivation Dwarfism. *Sci Am* 227: 76–82, 1972

Garfield, J. Social Stress and Medical Ideology. In CA Garfield (ed.): *Stress and Survival: The Emotional Realities of Life-Threatening Illness.* St. Louis: C.V. Mosby, 1979

Goffman, E. *Asylums.* New York: Doubleday, 1961

Gordon, G. *Role Theory and Illness.* New Haven: Yale University Press, 1966

Gore, S. The Effect of Social Support in Moderating the Health Consequences of Unemployment. *J Health Soc Behav* 19: 157–165, 1978

Harvey, JH (ed.). *Cognition, Social Behavior, and the Environment.* Hillsdale, NJ: Lawrence Erlbaum Associates, Publishers, 1981

Hebb, DO. *The Organization of Behavior.* New York: John Wiley, 1949

Henderson, S. The Social Networks, Social Support, and Neurosis: The Function of Attachment in Adult Life. *Br J Psychiatry* 13: 185–191, 1977

Henderson, S. A Development in Social Psychiatry: The Systematic Study of Social Bonds. *J Nerv Ment Dis* 168: 63–69, 1980

Henry, JP, and Stephens, PM. *Stress, Health, and the Social Environment: A Sociobiologic Approach to Medicine.* New York: Springer-Verlag, 1977

Hinkle, LE. Ecological Observations of the Relation of Physical Illness, Mental Illness, and the Social Environment. *Psychosom Med* 23: 289–297, 1961

Howard, H, and Scott, CA. Proposed Framework for the Analysis of Stress in the Human Organism. *Behav Sci* 10: 141–160, 1965

Jackson, CW, Jr, and Pollard, JC. Sensory Deprivation and Suggestion: A Theoretical Approach. *Behav Sci* 7: 332–342, 1962

Kalish, RA. Social Distance and the Dying. *Community Ment Health J* 2: 152, 1966

Kaplan, A. *Social Support: The Construct and Its Measurement.* B.A. Thesis, Department of Psychology. Providence, Rhode Island: Brown University, 1977

Kaplan, BH, Cassel, JC, and Gore, S. Social Support and Health. *Med Care* 15 (Supplement): 47–58, 1977

Kassebaum, GG, and Baumann, BO. Dimensions of the Sick Role in Chronic Illness. *J Health Soc Behav* 6: 16–27, 1965

Katz, AH. The Social Causes of Disease. In HP Dreitzel (ed.): *The Social Organization of Health.* New York: Macmillan, 1971, pp 5–14

King, IM. *A Theory for Nursing: Systems, Concepts, Process.* New York: John Wiley, 1981

Kornfeld, DS, Zimberg, S, and Malm, JR. Psychiatric Complications of Open-Heart Surgery. *N Engl J Med* 273: 287–292, 1965

Kosa, J, and Robertson, L. The Social Aspects of Health and Illness. In J Kosa, A Antonovsky, and I Zola (eds.): *Poverty and Health.* Cambridge, MA: Harvard University Press, 1969

LaRocco, JM, House, JS, and French, JRP, Jr. Social Support, Occupational Stress, and Health. *J Health Soc Behav* 21: 202–218, 1980

Lazarus, R. *Patterns of Adjustment.* New York: McGraw-Hill, 1976

Leff, HL. *Experience, Environment, and Human Potentials.* New York: Oxford University Press, 1978

Liem, JH, and Liem, R. Social Class and Mental Illness Reconsidered: The Role of Economic Stress and Social Support. *J Health Soc Behav* 19: 139–156, 1978

Lin, N, Simeone, RS, Ensel, WM, and Kuo, W. Social Support, Stressful Life Events, and Illness: A Model and an Empirical Test. *J Health Soc Behav* 20: 108–119, 1979

Ludwig, TD. Recent Marine Soils and Resistance to Dental Caries. In JB Bresler (ed.): *Environments of Man.* Reading, MA: Addison-Wesley, 1968, pp 45–51

Lynch, JJ. *The Broken Heart.* New York: Basic Books, 1977

Mechanic, D. The Concept of Illness Behavior. *J Chronic Dis* 15: 189–194, 1962

Merton, R. *Social Theory and Social Structure,* Revised edition. New York: The Free Press, 1968

Miller, P McC, and Ingham, JG. Friend, Confidents, and Symptoms. *Soc Psychiatry* 11: 51, 1976

Monteiro, L. After Heart Attack: Behavioral Expectations for the Cardiac. *Soc Sci Med* 7: 555–565, 1973

Moos, R, and Igra, A. Determinants of the Social Environments of Sheltered Care Settings. *J Health Soc Behav* 21: 88–98, 1980

Mueller, DP. Social Networks: A Promising Direction for Research on the Relationship of the Social Environment to Psychiatric Disorder. *Soc Sci Med* 14A: 147–161, 1980

Murdock, GP. *Theories of Illness: A World Survey.* Pittsburgh: University of Pittsburgh Press, 1980

Myers, JK, Lindenthal, JJ, and Pepper, MP. Life Events, Social Integration, and Psychiatric Symptomatology. *J Health Soc Behav* 16: 421–427, 1975

Myers, TI, Murphy, DB, and Smith, S. The Effect of Sensory Deprivation and Social Isolation on Self-Exposure to Propaganda and Attitude Change. *Am Psychol* 18: 440 (Abstract), 1963

Neuman, B. The Betty Neuman Health-Care Systems Model: A Total Person Approach to Patient Problems. In JP Riehl and SC Roy (eds.): *Conceptual Models for Nursing Practice.* New York: Appleton-Century-Crofts, 1980, pp 119–134

Newman, LF. Social and Sensory Environment of Low Birth Weight Infants in a Special Care Nursery: An Anthropological Investigation. *J Nerv Ment Dis* 169: 448–455, 1981

Newman, MA. *Theory Development in Nursing.* Philadelphia: F.A. Davis, 1979

Newman, MT. Ecology and Nutritional Stress in Man. In JB Bresler (ed.): *Environments of Man.* Reading, MA: Addison-Wesley, 1968, pp 104–116

Norbeck, JS. Social Support: A Model for Clinical Research and Application. *Adv Nurs Sci* 3, No. 4: 43–59, 1981

Norbeck, JS, Lindsey, AM, and Carrieri, VL. The Development of an Instrument to Measure Social Support. *Nurs Res* 30: 264–269, 1981

Parsons, T. *The Social Systems.* New York: The Free Press, 1951

Parsons, T. The Sick Role and the Role of the Physician Reconsidered. *Milbank Mem Fund Q* 53: 257–278, 1975

Patton, RG, and Gardner, LI. Deprived Dwarfism (Psychosocial Deprivation): Disordered Family Environment as Cause of So-called Idiopathic Hypopituitarism. In LI Gardner (ed.): *Endocrine and Genetic Diseases of Childhood and Adolescence.* Philadelphia: W.B. Saunders, 1975

Powell, GF, Brasel, JA, and Blizzard, R. Emotional Deprivation and Growth Retardation Simulating Idiopathic Hypopituitarism. 1. Clinical Evaluation of the Syndrome. *N Engl J Med* 276: 1271–1278, 1967

Prescott, JW. Somatosensory Affectional Deprivation (SAD) Theory of Drug and Alcohol Use. *Natl Inst Drug Abuse Res Monogr Ser* 30: 286–296, 1980

Read, M. *Culture, Health, and Disease.* London: Tavistock Publications, 1966

Renaud, M. On the Structural Constraints to State Intervention in Health. *Intl J Health Serv* 5: 559–571, 1975

Riehl, JP, and Roy, SC. *Conceptual Models for Nursing Practice,* Second edition. New York: Appleton-Century-Crofts, 1980

Riesen, AH, and Zilbert, DE. Behavioral Consequences of Variations in Early Sensory Environment. In AH Riesen (ed.): *The Developmental Neuropsychology of Sensory Deprivation.* New York: Academic Press, 1975, pp 211–252

Rogers, ME. *An Introduction to the Theoretical Basis of Nursing.* Philadelphia: F.A. Davis, 1970

Rogers, ME. Nursing: A Science of Unitary Man. In JP Riehl and SC Roy (eds.): *Conceptual Models for Nursing Practice,* Second edition. New York: Appleton-Century-Crofts, pp 329–337

Rossi, AM. General Methodological Considerations. In JP Zubek (ed.): *Sensory Deprivation: Fifteen Years of Research.* New York: Appleton-Century-Crofts, 1969, pp 16–43

Roy, SC. The Roy Adaptation Model. In JP Riehl and SC Roy (eds.): *Conceptual Models for Nursing Practice,* Second edition. New York: Appleton-Century-Crofts, 1980, pp 179–188

Roy, SC, and Roberts, SL. *Theory Construction in Nursing: An Adaptation Model.* Englewood Cliffs, NJ: Prentice-Hall, 1981

Salloway, JC, and Dillon, P. A Comparison of Family Networks and Friend Networks in Health Care Utilization. *J Comp Fam Stu* 1973: 131–142

Schneider, RA, Costiloe, JP, and Wolf, S. Arterial Pressures Recorded in Hospital and During Ordinary Daily Activities: Contrasting Data in Subjects with and without Ischemic Heart Disease. *J Chronic Dis* 23: 647–657, 1971

Scott, TH, Bexton, WH, Heron, W, and Doane, BK. Cognitive Effects of Perceptual Isolation. *Can J Psychol* 13: 200–209, 1959

Segall, A. *Sociocultural Variation in Illness Behavior.* Unpublished Ph.D. Dissertation. University of Toronto, 1972

Segall, A. The Sick Role Concept: Understanding Social Behavior. *J Health Soc Behav* 17: 163–170, 1976

Selye, H. Stress without Distress. In CA Garfield (ed.): *Stress and Survival: The Emotional Realities of Life-Threatening Illness.* St. Louis: C.V. Mosby, 1979, pp 11–16

Shannon, GW. Space, Time, and Illness Behavior. *Soc Sci Med* 11: 683–689, 1977

Stevens, BJ. *Nursing Theory: Analysis, Application, Evaluation.* Boston: Little, Brown, 1979

Suchman, E. Health Attitudes and Behavior. *Arch Environ Health* 20: 105, 1970

Suedfeld, P. Introduction and Historical Background; and Theoretical Formulations II. In JP Zubek (ed.): *Sensory Deprivation: Fifteen Years of Research.* New York: Appleton-Century-Crofts, 1969, pp 3–15; 433–448

Tees, RC, Midgley, G, and Bruinsma, Y. Effect of Controlled Rearing on the Development of Stimulus-Seeking Behavior in Rats. *J Comp Physiol Psychol* 94: 1003–1018, 1980

Townsend, JM. *Cultural Conceptions and Mental Illness: A Comparison of Germany and America.* Chicago: The University of Chicago Press, 1978

Turner, RJ. Social Support as a Contingency in Psychological Well-Being. *J Health Soc Behav* 22: 357–367, 1981

Twaddle, AC. *Influence and Illness: Definitions and Definers of Illness Behavior Among Older Males in Providence, Rhode Island.* Unpublished Ph.D. Dissertation. Providence, Rhode Island: Brown University, 1968

Twaddle, AC. Health Decisions and Sick Role Variations: An Exploration. *J Health Soc Behav* 10: 105–114, 1969

Twaddle, AC. *Sickness Behavior and the Sick Role.* Cambridge, MA: Schenkman Publishing Company, 1979

Urbach, P. Social Propensities. *Br J Philos Sci* 31: 317–328, 1980

Vaillant, GE. Natural History of Male Psychological Health: Effects on Mental Health and Physical Health. *N Engl J Med* 301: 1249–1254, 1979

Walker, KN, MacBride, A, and Vachon, MLS. Social Support Networks and the Crisis of Bereavement. *Soc Sci Med* 11: 35–41, 1977

Wapner, S, Cohen, SB, and Kaplan, B (eds.). *Experiencing the Environment.* New York: Plenum Press, 1976

Wilson, EO. *Sociobiology: The New Synthesis.* Cambridge, MA: Harvard University Press, 1975

Wolf, S. *Social Environment and Health.* Seattle, Washington: University of Washington Press, 1981

Wolf, S, and Goodell, H (eds.). *Stress and Disease,* Second edition. Springfield, IL: Charles C. Thomas, 1968

Wolff, G, and Money, J. Relationship Between Sleep and Growth in Patients with Reversible Somatotropin Deficiency (Psychosocial Dwarfism). *Am J Hum Genet* 25: 193–199, 1973

Wolinsky, FD, and Wolinsky, SR. Expecting Sick-Role Legitimation and Getting It. *J Health Soc Behav* 22: 229–242, 1981

Worrell, JD. Nursing Implications in the Care of the Patient Experiencing Sensory Deprivation. In CK Kintzel (ed.): *Advanced Concepts in Clinical Nursing.* Philadelphia: J.B. Lippincott, 1971, pp 130–143

Zubek, JP. Sensory and Perceptual-Motor Effects. In JP Zubek (ed.): *Sensory Deprivation: Fifteen Years of Research.* New York: Appleton-Century-Crofts, 1969, pp 207–253

Zuckerman, M. Hallucinations, Reported Sensations and Image; and Theoretical Formulations I. In JP Zubek (ed.): *Sensory Deprivation: Fifteen Years of Research.* New York: Appleton-Century-Crofts, 1969, pp 85–125; 407–432

# 6

# Theoretical Analysis of Phenomena in the Domain of Nursing Action

> Firstly, there is the unity in things whereby each thing is at one with it-
> self, consists of itself, and coheres with itself. Secondly, there is the
> unity whereby one creature is united with the others and all parts of
> the world constitute one world.
>
> *della Mirandola*

## OVERVIEW

This chapter presents theoretical ideas about phenomena of nursing and conceptualization of nursing action. The domain of nursing action is viewed as consisting of two distinct categories of conceptualization and theory: (A) the client-
nurse system for the client-nurse dyad phenomena; and (B) the nurse system for
the phenomena in the nurse as an actor of nursing actions.

The first section deals with the meanings of nursing action and presents the
rationale for adopting the differentiation of the domain into two conceptual
categories—the client-nurse system and the nurse system. The following section
is devoted to discussion of selected conceptual and theoretical models that apply
to a scientific study of phenomena from two separate orientations. Models for
nursing action in the client-nurse system are examined in terms of the models'
interactive or noninteractive orientation to nursing action and conceptualization
of nursing action and intervention. Discussions regarding the conceptualization

of nursing action in the nurse system focus on the need to develop systematic and theoretical ideas about the nature of phenomena in the nurse system as the nurse is practicing nursing. A separate section is devoted to discussions of issues related to the concept of nursing diagnosis. Recent developments in the area of nursing diagnosis make it necessary to focus on theoretical considerations for the concept and referrents of nursing diagnosis, as well as on the role of the concept in theory development in nursing.

The last section offers conceptual analyses of the phenomena of negotiation as an example of client-nurse system phenomena, and the phenomena of decision-making as an example of nurse system phenomena.

## MEANINGS OF NURSING ACTION

We now come to the core of what we are mainly interested in explaining, the central concern to nursing, for this domain embraces the elements that nursing as a discipline is made of. It involves what we do and how we perform those actions we call nursing.

As discussed in Chapters 4 and 5, many phenomena within humanity and the environment are of critical import to nursing; yet it is theoretical development for the domain of nursing action that is essential in order to elevate nursing to a scientific discipline. This is the domain to which theories of nursing belong as conceptual systems. Obviously, theoretical concerns for this domain are determined by a definition of nursing adopted in the study. If we consider nursing as a "particular way" of managing human health affairs, it is precisely this "particular way" that requires definition and by which relevant phenomena are identified for scientific explanation. Through scientific explanations of what goes on in the world of "nursing action," we are able to systematize our ways of acting and to prescribe specific actions to fit specific requirements. The ultimate objective of the science of nursing necessarily focuses on this ability to prescribe nursing actions.

In other words, our need to understand and explain scientific problems that reside in the domains of client and environment are for this ultimate purpose as well. More specifically, only those theoretical postulates and empirical questions that have ultimate significance for the contents of nursing action can be considered to be within the nursing frame of reference, and require scientific answers from the nursing angle of vision. The starting point, then, for a scientific study of nursing is in thinking of nursing activities as "purposive."

Nursing scientists have to be in a somewhat different position from that of pure scientists for whom detachment and debunking are, of necessity, essential attitudes toward their subject matters. While maintaining scientific objectivity and detachment, nursing scientists have to work in balance with the attitude of advocacy for "good practice." Indeed, the science of nursing is in finding ways to discard trivial and frivolous acts from the ordinary repertoires of what nurses perform in "doing nursing," and to replace these acts with interventions and therapies that have significant purpose and rationality.

In order to do this, it is necessary, first, to know (or find) ways of separating those nursing acts that are trivial or frivolous from those that are meaningful, in that they are "nursing" acts. Implied in this statement is an acceptance of the reality that all of what nurses do in ordinary nursing situations is not necessarily "nursing," and that nurses are neither sciential in all their acts nor able to make all their acts have nursing intentions. Although it is probably neither necessary nor possible to program (i.e., prescribe) every act of a nurse, that is, every act performed in a nursing situation, the essential objective for the science of nursing is to strive for a system of knowledge that will increase the percentage of rational and explained acts in the total repertoire of what the nurse does in nursing.

One primary way of arriving at this understanding is through deciphering the meanings of acts performed by nurses. This points us to an inductive method of study in which the description of the nursing world allows us to attach meanings to nursing acts and discover patterns of occurrence. For example, if we find that different nurses entering a terminally ill patient's room assume certain body postures and utter certain words to the patient, we would be in a position to question their meanings as well as effects on the patient. The inductive approach for the discovery of patterns and meanings of nursing acts is important for the science of nursing in its current developmental stage as a scientific field. This is not to say that the deductive approach is not useful for development in the science of nursing. Both approaches need to be applied appropriately in nursing.

## THE DOMAIN OF NURSING ACTION

There is an air of embarrassment in the nursing literature when it comes to defining nursing or nursing action in exact terms. Reluctance continues to exist in specifying what we mean by nursing action, although many nursing theorists are moving forward in theoretical development with tentative definitions.

Donaldson and Crowley (1978) indicate that nursing scholars generally are in agreement on what nursing should be concerned with, and Riehl and Roy (1980) found commonalities among five nursing models examined by them with respect to the characteristics of interventions prescribed as nursing. For example, they found that nursing interventions prescribed by these nursing models allow for the client's expression of feelings, are aimed at maintaining whatever independent behaviors are possible for the client, and provide new ways for increasing the client's independence (Riehl and Roy, 1980). Furthermore, there is a movement toward developing a common conceptual scheme for nursing, beginning with the works of the National Conference Group on Nursing Diagnosis. Nevertheless, a fuzziness still exists in conceptualization, especially in terms of defining the boundary within which actions are classified as nursing. This fuzziness can be attributed to the fact that most of what nurses do is not significantly different from what ordinary people do in their everyday lives. What is different is not the acts themselves, but when, how, and why they are carried out. In nursing, the same acts take on special meanings in their enactment.

A nurse sits with a dying patient as a wife sits with her dying husband. While the "act" of attending the last hours of a dying person may appear the same in these two occasions, the meanings of that act to the "attenders" and the client would be different, and the actual contents of the act of attending may be very different in a behavioral, affective, informational, and technical sense. Theoretical efforts in nursing, then, need to focus on how such ordinary actions take on professional, nursing meaning and in what ways they become different from ordinary human actions. In a nondeliberate effort to make nursing actions "unordinary," that is "technical," the current nursing world has become preoccupied with bringing into the core of nursing those actions that require competent use of technological instruments. Though this preoccupation results from the current use of technology in health care, technology has to be considered as *the tools of nursing,* not the content itself. The core of nursing actions resides in the human-to-human actions performed by a professional nurse for objectives that are oriented to the client's health-related affairs.

For theoretical thinking in this chapter, I propose a definition of nursing action as *behavior enacted by a person under the conscious aegis of "nursing."* Although this definition appears to be circular, the labeling of an act as "nursing" is necessary for both subjective and objective endorsement of the action in a social sense. Because nursing is a social role, the content of the role, i.e., the performance of it, has to be designated formally as belonging to that role. Since acts enacted in a given role may be different in many ways, it is difficult to describe the acts without enumerating every kind. It is more of a conceptualization issue rather than a definitional one to be concerned with what kinds of acts are of a nursing type.

By this way of thinking, then, nursing action takes on a specific meaning with respect to its locus of occurrence. It is this idea of locus that is used to differentiate nursing actions, as proposed in Chapter 3. The major differentiation of locus is made as (a) the client-nurse system and (b) the nurse system. Of course, this is not to negate many nursing actions that are carried out away from clients but on behalf of them, such as consulting with physicians, conferring with family members, or negotiating with referring agencies in behalf of the client. These certainly are behaviors that need to be included as appropriate nursing actions. My contention, here, is that the majority of nursing actions that are enacted outside of the client-nurse system belong in the nurse system at the conceptual level. I believe that such behaviors can be explained and predicted within the theoretical constructs for the nurse system phenomena.


## THE CLIENT-NURSE SYSTEM

Nursing actions in the client-nurse system occur in direct encounters between the client and the nurse. Conceptualization of what is happening in such encounters mainly depends on the scope with which specific phenomena are abstracted. Let us return to the last section of the scenario of Mr. Harold Smith that was presented in Chapter 3.

> Ms. Dumas, the nurse, enters the patient's room with the IV dose of cefamandole to be put through the IV line, and notices the uneaten dinner, signs of a quiet, depressed mood, and coughing. Mr. Smith's roommate is in a great deal of pain, having had abdominal surgery on the preceding day. He moans and groans aloud at times. Ms. Dumas administers the medication through the IV line and talks to Mr. Smith about his discomfort and coughing.

Each discrete act that occurs between Ms. Dumas and Mr. Smith can be conceived in a different phenomenal term in a particularistic mode of analysis. Thus, *exchange of mood, energy transfer, attentiveness,* etc., may be considered as particularistic concepts referring to some of the phenomena apparent in this situation. On the other hand, the occurrences in the situation may be conceptualized in a holistic posture, as *transaction, nurse-patient interaction,* or *therapeutic relationship*. Such differences in conceptualization of the phenomena apparently present in a nursing situation allow several levels of theoretical questioning, yet the locus of occurrence here remains on the level of client-nursing system.

Phenomena that occur between two individuals (sometimes more than two, especially when the client constitutes a group of people as a unit) who have come together into situations because one party is the client and the other the nurse are nursing phenomena, requiring understanding and explanation from the nursing perspective. Here it is necessary to differentiate nursing phenomena in the client-nurse system from those that are objects of explanation in other scientific fields. For example, a sociologist might consider the patterns of interaction between the nurse and the client as subject matter, properly so, for explanation within a theory of social exchange. The sociologist's focus is necessarily "social," and insofar as it remains to be conceived as social, it is a proper subject matter for a sociological explanation. The sociologist is interested in explaining their interaction in terms of how social norms, attitudes, and values influence interactional patterning; how interactions begin, develop, and terminate in such social situations; or how one party's use of social symbols affects others' reactions to them. These are valid and essential questions that sociology tries to answer in its proper relevance structure.

On the other hand, a nursing scientist may take the pattern of interaction between the nurse and the client as subject matter for explanation within a nursing theory. The nursing scientist focuses on understanding the phenomena with respect to how the nurse's behaviors influence the client's reactions to his or her health, problems, and health-care situations; what kinds of nursing behaviors in such interactions maintain the focus on the client; or what kinds of communicative patterns foster the client's learning of new health-care requirements. Nursing focus is apparent in such questions. The same world, then, is examined on two different planes, that is, from two entirely different perspectives, allowing postulations of scientific problems that are oriented to two different objectives: Sociology, in this case, is interested in furthering an understanding of human interaction as social phenomena, while nursing is interested in understanding nurse-client interaction as nursing intervention or as a part of nursing actions, and is directed toward a knowledge base that can enable prescriptions of most effective patterns of nursing behaviors in client-nurse exchanges.

What then are the valid criteria that can be used to point out those aspects of reality in the client-nurse system as appropriate for study from the nursing perspective? The valid criteria appear to rest with the kinds of questions that are posed in conceptualization. It is in the posture. The main question is this: *Would a variation of "this occurrence" (that is, any occurrence of a type) that is taking place between the client and the nurse in any way alter (or should alter) the way the client feels, perceives the world relevant to health, and proceeds to make future moves regarding his or her health state?* If the answer is yes, then you have successfully conceptualized a nursing phenomenon in the client-nurse system. In this way, nursing actions within the client-nurse system have two common characteristics:

1. They are actions "existentially" occurring in situations where a client and a nurse are present in respective roles.
2. They are actions of which goals are oriented manifestly in the client.

## THE NURSE SYSTEM

Nursing actions of the nurse system are rather vaguely defined in the literature. By definition, these are actions that are performed by nurses alone without the physical presence of a client or even with the physical presence of a client but not involving the client actively in the actions. Yet the goals of such actions are oriented to the client. These actions refer to intellectual or cognitive actions involved in providing nursing care to clients. The clearest example of such actions is what we call "nursing process." The concept of the nursing process refers to a set of intellectual actions performed by a nurse in systematizing actual nursing-care actions. The purpose of the nursing process and relevant features of the nursing process are inherently tied to the client's problems; nevertheless, the actions of the nursing process belong to the nurse system. As an actor, the nurse performs the following intellectually based activities within the process:

1. gathers information;
2. makes judgments about the nature of information available;
3. arrives at problem-statements based on many information networks;
4. examines available and possible kinds of strategies for the solution of problems;
5. selects certain types as appropriate and effective interventions;
6. carries out those interventions, adopting scientifically selected operational procedures;
7. evaluates outcomes of the intervention;
8. modifies the existing information-base on the client as well as the future *modus operandi* regarding the solution of the client's problems.

The nursing process is the most global way of conceptualizing nursing actions in the nurse system, for it includes nearly all aspects of nursing's intellectual processes. In a more particularistic approach, such phenomena as making nursing diagnosis, nursing problem-solving, nursing decision-making, prioritization in nursing, etc., may be considered appropriate concepts for scientific explanations.

As will be discussed in the later section in greater detail, theorizing for these classes of nursing action has not been extensive. Conceptualization of such phenomena as belonging to the general conceptual area of professional practice is rather new. The concept of "practice" including something other than what the nurse does with the client has been proposed by several authors in a general perspective (Bennis and Chin, 1976; Freidson, 1970; and Bourdieu, 1978). The concept of practice that refers to the cognitive aspects of professional actions, along with the behavioral and social aspects, appears to be a significant departure from earlier ideas about professional practice in which professionals are presumed to behave according to what they know. Variability in professional actions related to the professional's use of knowledge and cognitive processes that are used for translating "what one knows" to "what one does" is specifically at the core of questioning about the concept of practice. And it is precisely this notion that is vital to scientific study of nursing actions in the nurse system. This focus of theoretical questioning is not interested in "what" the nurse does with or for the client but in *"how the nurse arrives at given action choices."* There-

**TABLE 8. Examples of Concepts in the Domain of Nursing Action for Study in the Nursing Perspective**

| Domain Subsystem | Level of Concept Description | |
| --- | --- | --- |
| | Holistic | Particularistic |
| Client-nurse system | Caring | Exchange of mood |
| | Transaction | Liking |
| | Interaction | Hostility |
| | Therapeutic relation | Touch |
| | Agreement | Communication |
| | Attentiveness | Negotiation |
| | Influence | Empathy |
| | Comforting | Muscle condition-ing |
| | | Turning |
| | | Instructing |
| Nurse system | Nursing practice | Prioritization |
| | Expertise | Nursing assess-ment |
| | Nursing process | Decision-making |
| | Competence | Transference of experience |

fore, such phenomena rightly belong in the nurse system, although the goal-orientation of actions is in the client, not in the nurse.

Table 8 lists examples of concepts that are appropriate for scientific attention in this domain of nursing action according to two subsystems.

## MODELS FOR NURSING ACTION IN THE CLIENT-NURSE SYSTEM

All nursing theories and conceptual models include some notions about nursing action as defined from the perspective presented earlier, either explicitly or implicitly. The position of the nurse within the construct of nursing action fluctuates. Different nursing theorists consider and include the presence of the nurse in the enactment of nursing action with varying degrees of attention. At one extreme is the conceptualization of nursing action in which the nurse is simply the performer of nursing interventions. At the other extreme is the idea that the nurse's interactive presence is central to nursing intervention. Roy, Rogers, Orem, and Johnson consider the nurse's presence parenthetical to their main conceptualization of nursing intervention, whereas Peplau and King consider nursing actions from an interactive perspective. Mainly, the theoretical ideas of these six nursing theorists are discussed in detail in this section.

There are many other nursing models that may be categorized into these two camps, active (noninteractive) and interactive, according to their conceptualization of nursing actions, although they do not necessarily fit into one or the other category in a clear-cut way. In the first camp, Hall (1966) conceptualizes nursing action in terms of care and nurturing, not in an interactive sense but in an "active" sense on the part of the nurse. Wiendenbach (1964) also views nursing action as that directed to the client for whom actions as a helping process provide necessary requirements that will help restore the client's ability to cope with the demands of a healthy life. Neuman (1980) is similar to Roy in her conceptualization of nursing action. To Neuman, the purpose of nursing intervention is to reduce stress factors and adverse conditions that either affect or could affect optimal functioning of a client in a given situation. The inherent interactive, human, and professional qualities of the nurse are treated as givens in these models.

Orlando's conceptualization of nursing action, found in the second camp, is an interactional one in which the nurse's action is based on the client's reactions in situations of nursing care. The nursing action is thus viewed as a dynamic relationship (Orlando, 1961). Riehl's interaction model, based on symbolic interactionist orientation, conceptualizes nursing action as that of the nurse taking the role of the other in her relationships with the client (1980). Watson (1979) proposes that nursing action be based on "creative" factors and views the practice of caring as central to nursing. These conceptualizations adhere to the notion that nursing action is not simply doing things for the client or performing actions for the client, but involves the nurse as an interactive agent in a rather total way. Thus, the presence of the nurse according to this perspective is seen to be the central focus of nursing actions.

## Roy Adaptation Model

According to Roy, nursing interventions are activities that manipulate the client's focal, contextual, and residual stimuli in order to bring about the focal stimuli within the client's adaptation level (Roy and Roberts, 1981, p. 46). In this adaptation model, the phenomena of nursing action in the client-nurse system are conceptualized as nursing treatments for which human interactive processes may only be one form of treatment protocol rather than the treatment process itself. Roy's model suggests, therefore, that the variability of nursing action depends on "causes" for the client's inability to maintain a state of dynamic equilibrium, and that a nursing intervention is in the form of manipulating stimuli. The outcome of the nursing intervention (or dependent variable) is an alteration of the client's ineffective regulatory responses with respect to a specific aspect of the adaptive mode (Roy and Roberts, 1981). The following are examples of nursing action conceptualized, according to Roy and Roberts, as manipulation of stimuli:[1]

1. For the exercise and rest aspects of the physiological needs mode—positioning, conditioning exercises, joint mobility exercise, and environmental organization for the problem of immobility; minimizing of stimuli input and maintaining sleep rhythm for the problem of sleep deprivation.

2. For the temperature aspect of the physiological needs mode—altering environmental temperature, reducing physical activity, administering antipyretic drugs and measures, and administering dietary and fluid intake for the problem of hyperthermia; active or passive rewarming of the client for the problem of hypothermia.

3. For the senses aspect of the physiological needs mode—sensory stimulation, providing meaning for sensory stimulation and altering patterning of sensory stimulation for the problems of sensory deprivation or overload.

4. For nutrition, elimination, fluid and electrolytes, oxygen and circulation, and endocrine system aspects of the physiological needs mode—the objects of manipulation that are usually contextual stimuli for these subaspects in the physiological needs mode are defined in the model as fluid, activity, nutrition, communication, aeration, and pain. Therefore, nursing interventions for these aspects of adaptation involve maintaining fluid balance; reducing or increasing the client's activity in terms of physical, cardiopulmonary, metabolic or mental activity; adjusting dietary and nutritional supplements, including spiritual nutrients; allowing communication of fears; protecting the client from pulmonary aeration, manipulating environmental aeration, and allowing psychological aeration; alleviating both physical and psychological pain.

5. For the self-concept, role function, and interdependence aspects of psychosocial modes—assisting the client in role-taking; providing clear role cues; arranging for environmental changes that enhance a balance in nurturing and seeking nurturance.[2]

This listing indicates the conceptualization of nursing action in the Roy Adaptation Model as discrete activity. Nursing action is based on the nurse selecting appropriate contextual stimuli that are thought to impinge on the client's adaptation level, and then manipulating the stimuli by reducing, adding to, or changing the character of the stimuli. What this means is that nursing action is directed at causes that are making the client feel ill or be sick, rather than at the person as a whole who is experiencing a set of problems. Although the nurse is conceived as a set of contextual stimuli, manipulation of the nurse-self is only very superficially inferred in the conceptualization. The basic premise is that the nurse knows what is good for the client, and therefore should be able to perform manipulative activities dealing especially with the externally originating stimuli.

Since nursing action in the model is fundamentally directed toward "causes" of deviations from adaptive equilibrium, nursing interventions that are simply responding to the client's responsive states (for example, crying, thrashing about in bed, or appearing edematous) cannot be decided upon without an extraction of the causes for such behaviors. Thus, in an analytical sense, each nursing action needs to be directly linked to a specific aspect of the adaptive mode and to a set of specified contextual stimuli. The Roy Adaptation Model suggests the prescriptive connotation of nursing action directed toward a specific adaptive difficulty; yet the model (in the way it has been described so far) allows arbitrary selection of nursing interventions. In addition, the characteristics of nursing action take on many different forms, ranging from making arrangements of materials and information in the client's external world to actually impinging on the person physically. Therefore, in considering nursing action as an independent variable, it is necessary to identify a specific aspect of the adaptive mode as a dependent outcome. Hence, the goal of nursing action is "to promote patient adaptation with regard to the four modes—physiological needs, self-concept, role function, and interdependence—by changing the stimuli" (Roy and Roberts, 1981, pp. 44–45). However, the approach for nursing prescription is particularistic in that adaptation is treated for each mode separately.

## Rogers' Concept of Unitary Man

Rogers' conceptualization of nursing action is covertly done within the model of a unitary man. Rogers states that nursing practice is directed toward promoting symphonic interaction between a person and the environment, strengthening the coherence and integrity of the human field, and directing and redirecting patterning of the human and environmental fields for realization of maximum health potential (Rogers, 1970). For Rogers, nursing action is composed of behaviors, operations, and procedures, ranging from the use of instruments to human relationships. They are used with intellectual care in "rhythmic correlates of practice" in order to help people to achieve positive health or maximum health potential. The basic premises for nursing actions are (a) the wholeness of a person and his or her integrality with his or her environment, (b) the probabilistic patterning of individual evolution, and (c) the energy field as the fundamental, empirical unit of a person and the environment.

Health and illness are considered on a continuum, expressed according to the degree with which multiple events as a patterned influence affect the person's life processes at a given space-time. Because each human being is unique and whole, and since a person is conceived to have the capacity to reason and feel, and thus participates knowingly and probabilistically in the process of change, both the client and the nurse are integral participants in the nursing intervention process. The nurse, therefore, is an environmental component for the client, repatterning the energy field of the client's environment simply by being present. According to Rogers' model, nursing action, hence, is concerned with the following aspects:

1. Changing the client's values for probabilistic goal-setting that is responsive to the changing nature of the human and environmental fields. This involves the nurse realizing the client's individual potential and uniqueness for a future maturation relative to health.
2. Strengthening the person-environment resonancy by rearranging the rhythmic flow of energy waves between a person and his or her environment and by maintaining rhythmic consistency. This involves the nurse ordering or reordering the nature, amount, and speed of wave dispersion in the human and environmental fields for enhancement of the client's development relative to health.
3. Attaining the person-environment complementarity in an effort to acquire the best possible patterns of living coordinates for the client in coexistence with environmental changes. This requires the nurse to help the client come to terms with and realize individual differences and potentialities for directing change that are most beneficial to his or her evolution and the most effective fulfillment of life's capabilities.

These three categories of nursing action in Rogers' model suggest that nursing action is *not discrete activity but a process of holistic intervention.* Thus, the variability of nursing action can be expressed in qualitative terms rather than in nominative terms. Nursing action is conceptualized from the interactive perspective to the extent that the nurse's presence in the environment changes the characteristics of the environmental energy field and has the potential for strong influences on repatterning. The phenomena of mutual, complementary influence between the client and nurse is not distinctively conceptualized as a special case, for Rogers believes not in the human-to-human interaction as an essential phenomenon but in the human-to-environment interaction in which other individuals are quality-changing aspects of the environment as is the nurse.

Because nursing action is not directed at "solving" a health problem, the conceptualization of nursing action is not prescriptive. For that matter, the goal of nursing action is never deterministic. It is viewed in terms of "correlates" and mutual simultaneity. Hence, the outcomes of nursing action in the client are directed toward the more complex repatterning and organization of the energy field that are expected to occur in a probabilistic and correlative fashion, not in a cause-effect way.

## Orem's Self-care Model

Orem defines nursing as "a creative effort of one human being to help another human being" (1980, p. 55). Nursing action is conceptualized as a service to help another person in need of help by actions that are complementing or substituting for the actions of the person, or providing and fostering conditions to facilitate the development or exercise of the person's capabilities for self-care. Helping actions as compensatory or developmental services take the five forms identified by Orem (1980, pp. 61–68):

1. acting for or doing for another;
2. guiding another;
3. supporting another;
4. providing an environment that promotes personal development in relation to becoming able to meet present or future demands for action;
5. teaching another.

Each method is considered valid to the extent that it is used to maximize the "self-care agency" of the client, and this means that the variability of the nursing action method has to be aligned with the helping requirement level of the client.

Self-care action refers to human activity of a deliberate nature that is a goal-directed, result-seeking action. It is learned behavior that is acquired through knowledge, motivation, and skill. Since the nurse's client is conceived to be a person who is deficient in self-care agency, nursing actions are directed at compensating for and developing certain aspects of the client's self-care agency that are temporarily or more permanently lacking in terms of development, operability, and adequacy.

Accordingly, nursing action is a discrete action in two ways: a specific nursing action can be matched to a deficiency in the self-care agency in meeting particular self-care requisites, such as an inability to feed oneself; and a specific nursing action also assumes one of the five methodological characteristics of helping, such as guiding the client with the eating process. It is therefore prescriptive in nature as well as being discrete. Variability of nursing action in this model is both nominative and quantitative. Nursing action is conceptualized in the degree of the nurse's involvement in maintaining the self-care agency of the client and can be differentiated as three nursing systems: (a) a wholly compensatory nursing system in which the nurse is the principal performer of the client's self-care actions; (b) partly compensatory nursing system in which both the nurse and the client share in the performance of self-care actions; and (c) a sup-portive-educative nursing system in which the client requires development in order to be completely self-care competent. In addition, the nurse is the definer of nursing systems and is responsible for initiating, maintaining, and severing relationships with the client in a nursing system. The influence and control are seen as one-sided, residing with the nurse.

### Johnson's Behavioral System Model

Johnson (1980, p. 214) defines nursing action as "an external regulatory force which acts to preserve the organism and integration of the client's behavior at an optimal level under those conditions in which the behavior constitutes a threat to physical or social health, or in which illness is found." She further suggests that such external force may operate through the imposition of external regula-tory or control mechanisms, through attempts to change structural units in de-sirable directions, or through the fulfillment of the functional requirement of the subsystems. The nurse is there to "do" what is prescribed and appropriate for removing deleterious forces impinging on the client. Johnson thus also con-ceptualizes nursing action in a deterministic, discrete, and prescriptive manner. Within Johnson's behavioral system model, nursing action is directed toward establishing regularities in the client's behaviors identifiable on a subsystem level. Nursing actions may assume any of the four modes of intervention:[3]

1. Redirect behavior by imposing limits or controls over it or by sup-plementing or substituting immature or ineffective control mecha-nisms.
2. Defend structural integrity by providing protection from unneces-sary stressors and threats.
3. Inhibit irregular behaviors by suppressing ineffective responses.
4. Facilitate the establishment of new behaviors that are functional to the person by nurturance and stimulation.

The nurse either supplies a "sustenal imperative herself" or mobilizes other re-sources in carrying out nursing interventions selected among these four modes. For each mode of intervention, there are specific techniques from which the nurse makes a selection to be used in a given nursing situation.

These nursing models exemplify the conceptualization of nursing action from an *action* perspective rather than from an interactive perspective. The focus in these models is the nature of actions that are attributed to the nurse as "nurs-ing." Actions performed by the nurse are conceptualized to suggest variability as independent or dependent variables, depending on the focus of explanation. Conceptualizations of nursing action different from these models are offered by Peplau and King. Peplau and King view nursing action from an interactive per-spective and define "interaction" as having the focal quality of nursing.

## Peplau's Concept of Interpersonal Relation

Peplau defines nursing as a therapeutic, interpersonal process that helps the client solve problems and likewise moves the client toward the direction of creative, constructive, productive, personal, and community living (1962). To Peplau, nursing refers to relationships between the client and the nurse in which interactive processes become a maturing force and an educative instrument for both parties. Thus, although the principal aim of nursing is to guide the client toward new learning and a positive change for self-repair and self-renewal, the nurse also experiences growth and maturity through interpersonal involvement. Peplau conceptualizes the interpersonal process in four phases through which the client and the nurse attain therapeutic outcomes. Orientation, identification, exploitation, and resolution are the stages of interpersonal relations, of which nature, length, and effectiveness are determined not only by the nurse's ability to perform the roles of teacher, resource person, counselor, leader, technical expert, or surrogate, but also by the client's abilities and motivations for movement in the relationship. According to Peplau, the major variable characteristics that influence the outcome of the interpersonal process are (a) the sequentiality of the interpersonal relation and (b) the nature of efforts of both actors in their collaborativeness or independence.

Independent variables that prescribe the need for the interpersonal process are psychobiological conditions such as needs, frustration, conflict, or anxiety that are detrimental to an individual's maturing process. Outcomes of nursing action as interpersonal process are oriented to the total person rather than to specific aspects of the individual. The most significant departure in Peplau's ideas of nursing action from those developed by others is in the recognition that experiential growth from the interaction takes place not only in the client but also in the nurse. A resulting postulation is that a nurse will become increasingly proficient and effective in interpersonal relations with clients as the nurse's experiences in nursing action increase. However, this conceptualization does not consider the applicability of interpersonal process as a holistic modality of nursing action for a variety of problems a client may present and is limited in that way.

## King's Model of the Interpersonal System
## (Theory of Goal Attainment)

King's idea of nursing is based on the conceptualization of the nursing system as comprised of dynamic interacting systems. Within the dynamic interacting personal, interpersonal, and social systems, nursing occurs as actions, reactions, and interactions through which information is shared, relationships are created between the nurse and the client, and goals and the means for attaining the goals for the client's health are mutually established (King, 1981).

According to King, interactional aspects of nursing action accordingly encompass actions of perceiving, thinking, relating, judging, and acting against the behavior of individuals who come to a nursing situation. The client-nurse interaction, the dyad interaction, is one type of interpersonal system in which several processes of the system are used to attain a goal. The processes can be summarized as follows (King, 1981):

1. Perception—process used to attain information about each other and the situation.
2. Communication—process for exchange and interpretation of information that each imparts in the interaction.
3. Transaction—process of sharing values, needs, and wants through interaction.
4. Role—process by which the nature of the relationship and modes of communication to be used in the relationship are identified.
5. Stressor—process of becoming energy responses to the other.

These are expressible in variable terms to indicate the quality of nursing. Dependent variables of nurse-client interaction are goal attainment for the client, satisfaction, and enhancement of growth and development. Relationships among the different processes of interaction are hierarchical in that the perceptual process precedes communication, and both perception and communication affect the transaction. At the same time, the processes of role and stressor influence all other aspects of interaction. King's model considers interaction as a descriptive, yet normative process, oriented to the client in a holistic way. Interaction is the fundamental mode of nursing action from which all other subsequent actions and transactions evolve for the attainment of goals.

As shown in these summaries, conceptualizations of nursing action from the client-nurse system perspective vary greatly in their orientations in an action/interaction focus, with respect to the level of goal specificity (i.e., discrete/global), and in terms of prescriptive versus experiential orientation. Theoretical explanations of the phenomena of nursing action from this perspective may take on various analytical forms as well. Nursing action may be a discrete activity performed in order to correct some deviation in the client. In contrast, it may be the immersion of two individuals, a client and a nurse, in a total experience of interaction. Even at such extremes, the goal is always directed toward the client, any unexpected as well as expected changes in the nurse notwithstanding.

## MODELS FOR NURSING ACTION
## IN THE NURSE SYSTEM

Conceptualization of nursing action in the nurse system is rarely done by nursing theorists in a systematic way. Most models treat the aspects of nursing action in the nurse system as natural occurrences. Otherwise, it is considered to be encompassed within the idea of nursing process that the profession has come to accept as a universally correct *modus operandi* for providing nursing care. During the last two decades, nursing process has become well incorporated into the nursing knowledge system, and is considered the systematic way of giving care. The American Nurses Association's Standards for Practice are based on this form of problem-solving and action in nursing. Nursing process as an accepted "theory" or "principle" for provision of nursing care is treated by most nursing theorists in their writings as such. Application of the nursing model in the nursing process is discussed in great detail in many writings.[4]

The attitude that nursing action follows naturally from nursing assessment is particularly prominent in models in which nursing action is viewed in a prescriptive manner. For example, according to the Roy Adaptation Model, the nurse knows what to do if the behavior of the client has been clearly specified, linking it to its predominant stimuli in the nurse's assessment, since the "intervention is based specifically on the nursing assessment" (Roy and Roberts, 1981, p. 47). Further on, they state that:

> Based on this model [the Roy Adaptation Model], some nursing interventions will be traditional techniques such as comfort measures or health teaching. However, our theoretical work may allow us to discover entirely new activities that are the unique responsibility of the nurse when she is viewed as the promoter of patient adaptation.[5]

What they do not consider "problematic" in these statements is "how a nurse will discover a new activity," or "how a nurse makes a choice of a new activity over an old one," or even "why a nurse might want to seek new activities." In this model, the nurse is required to make "judgments" about ineffective processes influencing the client's adaptation level in order to come up with a diagnostic label for an ineffective behavior. It is exactly this phenomenon of nursing judgment that is problematic when a nurse scientist shifts the focus from the client to the nurse. The phenomenon of nursing judgment is an example of constructs that belong to nursing action in the nurse system, requiring scientific explanations.

Similarly, Neuman (1980) considers the use of the assessment/intervention tool designed according to the Neuman Health Care System model to offer a prescriptive base for nursing action. Like Roy, Neuman views the selection of nursing action as deterministic upon the adoption and careful use of an assessment tool.

Johnson (1980) also views the use of the behavioral system model in nursing process as the prescriptive, deterministic base for selecting and carrying out nursing interventions. Analysis of data regarding problematic behaviors leads to categorically and individually identified diagnosis, which in turn indicates the nature of the nursing problem. Identification of the nursing problem then directs the nurse to select the method of nursing intervention, which is arrived at through the clarification of focus of nursing action and identification of approach.

Rogers is somewhat more specific and states that professional nursing practice is creative and imaginative, and is considered to be rooted in "abstract knowledge, intellectual judgement, and human compassion" (Rogers, 1970, p. 122). She believes that nursing action is not determined by set formulas, and that the nurse's ability to select appropriate tools of practice is an intellectual skill. Rogers identifies three variables as those influencing the safe practice of nursing (i.e., how the nurse selects appropriate actions and how selected actions are put together): (a) the nature and amount of scientific knowledge, (b) the imaginative, intellectual judgment, and (c) human compassion.

> Intellectual skill in selecting those tools and procedures best suited to a given situation and artistry in utilization of mechanical and personal resources are important dimensions of nursing practice. However, it must be thoroughly understood that tools and procedures are adjuncts to practice and are safe and meaningful only to the extent that *knowledgeable nursing judgements underwrite their selection and the ways in which they may be used*.[6]

She continues:

> Nursing practice must be flexible and creative, individualized and socially oriented, compassionate and skillful. Professional practitioners in nursing must be continuously *translating theoretical knowledge into human service* and participating in the coordination of their knowledge and skills with those of professional personnel in other health disciplines.[7]

Although these are pointed out as essential elements for good nursing practice, Rogers does not follow through with the idea in her model. Conceptualization in which an explanation of variable conditions of such phenomena as "translating knowledge" or "using the tools of practice" in the nurse system is not offered in the model of unitary man. Theoretically, Rogers' statements are rhetorical and fall short of scientific explanation. While she identifies phenomena requiring scientific explanation, she neither offers exact definitions of elements critical for variations in the nurse's actions nor describes the way these elements are related to each other and related to the contents of nursing action.

King's notion of nursing practice in the nurse system is incorporated into the concept of give-and-take, the interaction that is the basis for nursing decision-making in the model (1981). Thus, the variables influencing nursing action in the nurse system are what the nurse brings into the client-nurse interaction situation. These are the nurse's perceptions, skills in communication, values for transaction, role-concepts, and stress. Identical elements in variable forms are also brought into the interaction by the client. Nursing action varies not because of what the nurse processes in isolation from the client, but only as a result of the nature of the interactional evolution that takes place with what the nurse and the client bring into the situation and how they work together. This suggests that King considers phenomena of nursing action on only one analytical plane. Nursing action as a process does not exist in the nurse system; the nurse is a variable for nursing action for what the nurse is and how she or he participates in interaction.

In a more specific fashion, Orem (1980) proposes the concept of *nursing agency,* denoting the nurse's specialized abilities. Nursing agency includes (a) specialized education, (b) specialized knowledge of the nursing situation, (c) mastery of technology of nursing practice, and (d) motivation for practice. The characteristics of nursing action in the nurse system are expressed in terms of the art of nursing and nursing prudence. The art of nursing means creating systems of nursing assistance and care, and depends upon the quality of the nurse for creative investigations and analyses and syntheses of information within the nursing situation. On the other hand, nursing prudence means rightly doing selected acts in a given situation based on one's knowledge of the situation. It depends on that quality of a nurse that is related to the ability to seek and take counsel in new or difficult nursing situations, to make correct judgment for action under changing conditions, to decide to act in a particular way, and to take action. The art of nursing and nursing prudence are influenced by experience primarily, but interactively also by such variables as a nurse's talent, personality, developed and preferred modes of thinking, stages of personal and moral development, ability to conceptualize complex situations of action and to analyze and synthesize information, and life experiences (Orem, 1980).

Thus, according to Orem's conceptualization of nursing practice, an activated nursing agency produces nursing operations and actions that vary in terms of the art of nursing and nursing prudence. The basic postulation is that nursing agency, in combination with other personal characteristics of the nurse, influences the nature and mastery of those nursing actions performed. This model, however, does not deal with the issue of *how* nursing actions are selected and performed in certain ways by the nurse. Orem conceptualizes the phenomena of nursing actions in the nurse system in a holistic manner.

These are beginning conceptualizations of many aspects of nursing actions in the nurse system. It appears that there are two distinct approaches to conceptualizing nursing action in the nurse system, as there are in other domains. The first approach is a holistic one by which the total process is perceived as *nursing practice* or *nursing process.* The second approach is a particularistic mode by which many phenomena are distinctly perceived as separate concepts such as decision-making, prioritization, improvisation, problem-solving, nursing diagnosis, transfer of knowledge, etc.

Conceptualization of nursing action in the nurse system either in the holistic or the particularistic approach points up two variable characteristics of the phenomena: quality of nursing action and methodological difference in nursing action. Hence, for example, the phenomena of the nursing process can be considered for scientific explanation with respect to the qualitative nature (e.g., good/bad; effective/ineffective; or efficient/inefficient), and to the techniques of adoption (e.g., sequential application; frequency of use; time of use; independent/team approach). Nursing decision-making can also be thought of in these two ways: (a) good/bad, appropriate/inappropriate, or adequate/inadequate, which are qualitative aspects of the decision-making, regardless of actual techniques adopted in the process; and (b) adoption of specific techniques of decision-making such as optimization, "satisficing," or balance techniques.

Two sets of variables may be linked to the phenomena of nursing action in the nurse system: One set is exogenous to the nurse system, and the other is inherent in the nurse system. Exogenous variables that may influence such phenomena are organizational structure and force of nursing care, nursing service structure, the client's nursing care requirements, peer support, climate of nursing care, etc. For example, the quality of the nursing process as carried out by a nurse is partly influenced by the normative expectations apparent in the nursing service setting, the amount of actual as well as perceived time available to the nurse to systematize the nursing care, and the complexity of nursing care requirements presented to the nurse by clients. Organizational and external stresses have been attributed to less-ideal provisions of nursing care and to the phenomenon of "reality shock" in new graduates.

On the other hand, the way a nurse carries out nursing action is also affected by many factors inherent in the nurse. The nurse's knowledge level, educational preparation, intellectual skill, personality, past experiences, world view, and feeling states affect the "quality" of nursing action. Wrong decisions are made because of the way the nurse evaluates the situation, or because the nurse has a limited experience with specific life and nursing situations with which he or she can develop evaluative frameworks.

This questioning suggests a need for theoretical or conceptual models that describe and explain the phenomena of nursing action in the nurse system and relationships among different components identified as relevant for the study, as shown in Figure 4. The subject matter for such theoretical orientation is different from that which is dealt with in nursing models that are aimed at describing and explaining the phenomena in the client domain, and are directed toward nursing intervention prescriptions.

The uncertainty that is inherent in nursing practice is another area of importance for scientific explanation. The uncertainty in nursing practice is parallel to that found in medical practice (Fox, 1957; Merton, 1976; and Coser, 1979), and refers especially to uncertain outcomes of nursing interventions. However, the uncertainty in nursing practice is also present in making assessments about a client's presenting problems. Apparent interactions among physiological, psychological, and cognitive aspects of human responses produce complex phenomena in the client, making it rather difficult to make cause-effect linkages in a nursing assessment.

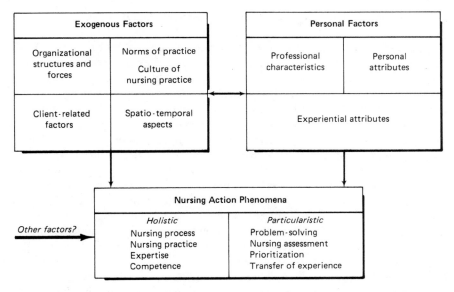

*Figure 4.* Factors for scientific study of the nurse system in the domain of nursing action.

Even though the prescriptiveness in the way nursing interventions are recommended for different client problems in several nursing models is suggestive of the deterministic nature of nursing practice, the practice implications of any prescription remain uncertain in judgment as well as in outcome. Thus, actual and potential uncertainty in nursing practice may influence the behavioral patterns of the nurse. Grier and Schnitzler (1979) examined the nurse's risk-taking behaviors in decision-making, and found that a nurse's propensity to take risk is related to the nature of the decision-making situation as well as the nurse's educational level. Nursing decisions are uncertain to the extent that the outcomes of decisions are probabilistic or multifactorially complicated and that the decisions themselves are based on incomplete information. Such uncertainty will, in turn, influence the nurse's actual decision-making and practice behaviors.

In this section, nursing action is considered from the perspective of the nurse system, focusing on nursing practice phenomena that are present within the nurse as an acting person. The discussions suggest a need for a careful delineation of conceptual differences between nursing action of the client-nurse system and that of the nurse system. A unique body of knowledge is needed to explain not only what we do in nursing for and with the client, but also how we do it.

## ISSUES IN THE CONCEPT OF NURSING DIAGNOSIS

The discussions offered in the preceding sections of this chapter bring us to conceptual issues regarding the concept of nursing diagnosis. The reasons for dealing with the concept in a separate section are two-fold: In a definitional sense, nursing diagnosis is a label that is attached to a phenomenon (or a cluster of phenomena) present in a client, indicating that the phenomenon requires a nursing solution. Thus, the naming of client phenomena has to depend in the first place on the way "client" is conceptualized, and secondly, on the definition of a nursing solution vis-a-vis a medical solution, or pharmacological solution, or social service solution, etc. In addition, a nursing diagnosis as a phenomenon is a "created" phenomenon. A nurse has to perform a labeling act in examining the reality that is present in the client and by selecting relevant facts. Nursing diagnosis is a way of translating "natural phenomena" to have specific, scientific "nursing" meanings. It is a systematic conceptualization of phenomena in the client system from a nursing perspective, not only for descriptive understanding, but necessarily for prescriptive purposes. Nursing diagnosis is necessary only because one is interested in also making decisions about a specific nursing solution (or what is also termed as nursing intervention, nursing approach, or nursing therapy).

In accepting the nursing process as the major scientific approach for delivering nursing service during the past two decades, the nursing profession has also basically accepted the concept of nursing diagnosis as a process through which a nurse arrives at a judgment regarding the client's problems requiring a nursing solution. However, there still is an interchange in the use of terms—nursing diagnosis, nursing problems, nursing needs. Whether or not a nurse comes up with an exact name for the client's problem in nursing terms, the diagnosing act for the nurse has been included firmly and formally in the nursing process. In general, nursing theorists, nursing researchers, and nursing practitioners agree that a nurse, in delivering a systematic, scientific nursing service to the client, should go through the step of identifying the client's problems and arriving at a list (i.e., nursing problem statement, list of nursing needs, or nursing diagnosis) that is then scrutinized for a nursing solution. Therefore, the controversies are not related to the basic concept of nursing diagnosis. The major issues are related to (a) varying views regarding "clinical" referents of nursing diagnosis, and (b) nursing diagnosis classification system.

## REFERENTS OF NURSING DIAGNOSIS

It is generally accepted that nursing diagnosis refers to health problems or health states that are treated by means of nursing intervention (Gebbie and Lavin, 1975; Lash, 1981). Health problems that are the referents of nursing diagnosis have been conceptualized from nursing perspectives in a variety of ways. As an attempt to differentiate nursing diagnosis from medical diagnosis, Aspinall (1978) views health problems in nursing diagnosis as impaired body functions, while several others (Durand and Prince, 1966; and Roy, 1975) view health problems in terms of responses to illness or pathological conditions. Gordon (1976) identifies health problems in terms of signs and symptoms. Jones (1979), on the other hand, states that a nursing diagnosis is the statement of a person's responses to a situation or illness that is actually or potentially unhealthful and that a nursing intervention can help to change in the direction of health, a concept adopted from Mundinger and Jauron (1975).

The definition proposed by the theorists at the Third National Conference is more global: "Nursing diagnosis is a concise phrase or term summarizing a cluster of empirical indicators representing patterns of unitary man."[8] Although this definition has been developed by a group of nursing theorists and suggests general agreement in viewing problems of human health, the actual application of this definition in "creating" conceptual labels (or terminologies) for nursing diagnostic states is at variance with the concept of wholeness. In addition, nursing theoretical models already developed have their own definitions of health problems: adaptation (Roy), self-care deficit (Orem), patterns of unitary man (Rogers), responses to stressors (Neuman), and behavior (Johnson). As indicated by Gordon (1979), there is a lack of consensus on the referents of nursing diagnosis.

There is general acceptance of the idea that nursing diagnosis does not (or should not) refer to pathological deviations or disease states. However, nursing diagnosis may refer to health problems and health states focusing on many different aspects of human experience. Stevens lists the following five examples (1979, p.95):

1. experiential states,
2. physiologic deviations from the norm,
3. problematic behaviors,
4. altered relationships,
5. reactions of others.

Stevens' observation was based on the list established by the National Conference Group's work. This group's continuing efforts as well as others' work oriented to establishing a "complete" list seem to bring forth more confusion in specifying the exact characteristics or criteria of referents of nursing diagnosis. For example, Avant (1979) developed a set of criteria for nursing diagnosis of maternal attachment. In proposing this as a nursing diagnosis, Avant submitted a vast array of nonproblematic phenomena as possible referents for nursing diagnosis. Indeed, this is philosophically correct, since nursing is concerned with enhancement of health and healthful behavior. However, making diagnosis about nonproblematic phenomena raises a question of suitability: Should the nursing diagnosis indicate the results of differentiation and abstraction of problems that require nursing attention? Or should the nursing diagnosis indicate concise statements descriptive of human conditions? The question also is how rigorously should we follow the criteria for rejection: ''Any rejection [of a category from the list of nursing diagnoses established by the National Conference Group] should be based on clinical evidence that the diagnosis provides no basis for nursing intervention.''[9]

The general statement accepted by the theorists at the Third National Conference appears to reflect the second position, that nursing diagnosis is a term denoting a description of a human condition. However, the diagnostic nomenclature approved by the Group includes only problematic phenomena, denoted by such terms as *alterations in, impairment of, abnormal, dysfunctional, inadequate, lack of,* and *disturbance in* (Kim and Moritz, 1982). These refer to deviated and problematic states in *structural* (i.e., alteration, lack, disturbance, and inadequacy) and *functional* (impairment, abnormality, and dysfunction) aspects of human phenomena. In addition, the list also includes areas of diagnosis related to the *process* aspect of human phenomena, such as grieving, coping, or manipulation. This observation calls attention to the need to develop conceptual systems that may be used to point out referents of nursing diagnosis. Of course, as pointed out by Stevens (1979), it is related to the problem of defining the subject matter for nursing and nursing practice. Therefore, specifying the referents of a nursing diagnosis is closely linked to the conceptualization of phenomena in the domain of client.

## NURSING DIAGNOSIS CLASSIFICATION SYSTEM

The impetus for development of a classification system of nursing diagnosis has culminated from the positions that ''without such a system, nurses will continue to experience difficulty in educating beginning practitioners, designing and performing research, and communicating nursing care within the nursing profession or across the health system,''[10] and that ''the development of a diagnostic classification system for nursing is an essential next step in the development of the science of nursing.''[11] These positions are congruent with the ideals and hopes of the profession, and seem to suggest a diagnostic classification system as a way of defining the content of nursing's subject matter. This attempt is also thought of as a step in theory development in nursing (Henderson, 1978; Kritch, 1979; and Roy, 1975). Kritch (1979) believes a nursing diagnosis classification system is a factor-isolating theory on which the next level of theory development is based.

The National Conference Group has adopted the inductive approach of what they termed a taxonomic classification of nursing diagnosis (Gebbie,

1975). By adopting the inductive method, the Group bypassed the question of "theoretical orientation" of the classification system, their later adoption of the conceptual framework of unitary man notwithstanding. Their position is to arrive at an agreement on the *problem-label, etiology,* and *signs and symptoms,* i.e., *defining characteristics* for diagnostic categories by using language that is not theory-based. By being atheoretical in its approach, the classification system may be accepted, tested, and used by nurses with different theoretical orientations. However, a conceptual system that is composed of a definition, a causal statement as to why such phenomenon occurs (etiology), and operationalization of the term (defining characteristics) cannot be derived without theoretical premises. It appears, then, that a classification system developed in a manner such as adopted by the National Conference Group is multitheoretical rather than atheoretical.

Another question is related to the implications of a nursing diagnosis classification system for nursing intervention. Would such a system result in nursing's own version of Merck's Manual? To what extent will the nursing diagnosis nomenclature dictate nursing intervention prescriptions? And to what extent would alternative classification systems of diagnostic terms that are based on specific nursing theories be accepted and used interchangeably with other systems? Could a unified nomenclature of nursing diagnosis classification incorporate alternate "explanations of etiology" that are based on other theoretical assumptions and postulations? These are questions nursing scientists and practitioners should deal with and debate if we are not to be stifled by "a need to have a system," and if we are to allow multiple approaches to theoretical development in nursing.

## SELECTED CONCEPTUAL ANALYSES

As have been presented in Chapters 4 and 5, two concepts are examined in this chapter as examples of phenomena in the Domain of Nursing Action. The concept of *negotiation* is presented as an example of nursing action phenomena in the client-nurse system, and the concept of *nursing practice* is analyzed as an example of nursing action phenomena in the nurse system. As stated in the earlier chapters, the main purpose of this section is to show how a first-level analytical approach is used to gain conceptual and empirical understanding of phenomena within the domain of nursing action. Each concept is analyzed with respect to (a) definitional clarification and conceptual meanings as reflected in the literature, (b) measurement and operationalization of concepts as a step toward an empirical analysis, and (c) the concept's relationships with other concepts that are important in nursing. The strategy and rationale for the conceptual analysis were discussed in detail in Chapter 2, and that rationale is adopted in this section for the analyses of negotiation and nursing practice.

## NEGOTIATION IN NURSING

Negotiation between the nurse and the client as a phenomenon of nursing action has been most frequently discussed in relation to patient compliance. Yet, negotiations are found in various nursing situations for some kinds of outcomes occurring in informal, incidental ways as well as in a formal fashion. An informal, incidental negotiation may be found in a nurse-client exchange. For example, a nurse prods and cajoles a client who is in surgical pain to ambulate while the client implores and pleads against it, and yet afterwhile they find a solution together that is agreeable to both, a negotiation. A formal negotiation in nursing may be found in contingency contracting in which the nurse and the client come to terms regarding the desired or targeted new behavior in the client and the reward in exchange for performance of that behavior, as described by Swain and Steckel (1981).

Negotiation in nursing analyzed in this section only refers to negotiation between nurse and client, rather than client and family, nurse and nurse, or nurse and physician. Although such negotiations occur in nursing, these are not central to the nursing action perspective of the client-nurse system.

### Definition

As stated in Webster's dictionary, *negotiation* is a conferring, discussing, or bargaining to reach an agreement in a generic sense, and it requires two parties, individuals or groups, in order for the phenomenon to occur. Strauss accepts the concept of negotiation as one of the possible means of "getting things accomplished" when two or more parties need to deal with each other to get those things done (1978). Negotiation occurs as individuals involved in an interaction attempt to attain certain consequences or outcomes that are realizable only through dealings with another party or parties.

Negotiation may be oriented to many different kinds of consequences, some tangible such as labor contracts, and others intangible such as general understanding of each other's position or rules of behavior. Since negotiations take on different characteristics according to specific structural conditions of interaction, i.e., parties (persons), context (time and situation), and subject, negotiations in nursing are special cases of a general type in this respect.

Several characteristics differentiate negotiations in nursing from a general type. First, negotiations in nursing are between two parties having specific social roles, those of nurse and client, and occur in interactions characterized by these role-relationships. Second, negotiations in nursing occur in health-care situations, in which most clients are more or less "captive," in the sense that they are restricted from walking away freely from the situations. Third, negotiations in nursing are oriented to consequences that are aimed at the client's benefits. Therefore, motivation for negotiation on the part of the nurse is assumed to be inherently "selfless" and other-oriented (i.e., client-oriented).

Negotiation in nursing is a rather new concept. Traditionally, clients and professionals are considered to have a one-sided relationship in which the distribution of power and knowledge between the two parties is unequal. Freidson's classical analysis of professional dominance in medicine indicates the use of power and expertise in influencing the patient's vulnerability (1970). In recent years, however, there has been a growth of popular discussions about the role of the client in influencing the nature of the health-care that one receives. With the emerging realization among health-care professionals that clients possess resources that can be used to recover and maintain health, and that the client's passivity in health-care probably is not conducive to optimal health-care outcomes, collaborative models of professional practice have been proposed in various forms. In nursing, involvement of clients in their care has been a long-standing value, and has been emphasized more strongly in recent years along with the concepts of primary nursing and self-care. However, the processes by which negotiations occur in nursing and the nature of negotiations in nursing have not been conceptualized formally, nor have they been formally incorporated into nursing practice protocols.

Negotiation is a reciprocal, dynamic exchange between the nurse and the client in an effort to arrive at a mutually acceptable solution through a balanced use of expert knowledge, power, human sensitivity, and understanding. As a process, it is interactional and follows a sequence. The sequence of negotiation starts with an initial approach of two parties (a nurse and a client), in which a recognition of the need for reconciliation or bargaining occurs. Exchange-encounters, in which an option in solutions is not available or permitted, preempt the possibility of them advancing to negotiations.

From the initial state, the process of negotiation becomes diversified in its form and content according to the following six attributes, as described by Zartman (1976) and Strauss (1979):

1. the parties' previous experiences and encounters;
2. patterns and outcomes of previous negotiations between the parties;
3. distribution of actual and perceived power between the parties;
4. the values and costs at stake to both parties;
5. expertise in the use of negotiation techniques;
6. personal attributes used for influencing each other.

The final stage of the process culminates in the nature of negotiation outcomes that may be differentiated according to (a) outcomes' temporal limits, i.e., how long the agreement resulting from a specific negotiation is binding to the parties; (b) manifest and latent (tacit) meanings of the agreement; and (c) applicability and transferability of the agreement to other situations or its generalizability.

In nursing, then, negotiations occur when the nurse and the client realize difference(s) in opinions, approaches, or solutions regarding the client's nursing care. Negotiations may involve the goal of nursing care, the type of nursing care or procedures in nursing, and self-care. Negotiations in nursing may be oriented to solving conflicts that are only inherent in one specific situation or that have long-range implications, especially when they are related to lifestyle behaviors or long-term goals.

### Operationalization

Negotiation as it refers to a process is difficult to operationalize. A descriptive operationalization, at best, indicates the nature of negotiation. Because the process of negotiation is viewed to be influenced by the six structural aspects identified above, the actual operationalization needs to be made outside of these factors. Negotiation has been operationalized in terms of the time it takes to arrive at an agreement, the qualitative change that exists in the final agreement from the original wishes of both parties, and forms of interactional exchange used during the process, especially in terms of communication patterns.

In most studies of negotiation the units of analysis are: (a) whether or not negotiation is present in a situation, (b) how long a negotiation session lasts, or (c) what results from a negotiation session. Qualitative operationalization in terms of good/bad, effective/ineffective, or promotive/destructive, has not often been considered.

### Relationships with Other Concepts

Zartman (1976) summarizes seven different approaches used in the literature to explain outcomes of negotiation:

1. evolutionary explanation,
2. contextual explanation,
3. structural explanation,
4. strategic explanation,
5. personality explanation,
6. behavioral explanation,
7. process explanation.

These seven approaches of explanation identify variables that influence or determine outcomes of negotiation. In nursing, the following may be applicable variables for studying negotiations according to these seven approaches.

*1. Effects of formality of negotiation.*    It appears that formalized negotiation in nursing forces both the nurse and the client to enter into the process, while parties involved in informal negotiation may escape from the process without coming to agreements when the process becomes uncomfortable or stressful. Effects of delay or interruption may be significant for the provision of nursing care. Since there are no formal sanctions that either force or prescribe negotiated order in the client-nurse interaction, the form of negotiation in nursing should be considered in terms of client-care outcomes.

*2. Influence of the context of nursing care.*   Contexts in which the nurse and client come together for negotiation vary according to type of health-care organization (ambulatory, acute care, long-term care, or home), type of nursing service system (for example, primary nursing or team nursing), power distribution, organizational philosophy, etc. Physical and ecological contexts may have influence on certain types of negotiations in clinical settings.

*3. Effect of the structure of the relationship.*   Although tied to the contexts in many ways, structures of nurse-client relationships refer to the patterns of communication and influence. Such factors as role-orientations of the nurse and the client and their evaluations of the relationships will influence the outcomes of negotiations.

*4. Effect of strategic elements.*   Contingency contracting is a form of negotiation used in nursing in which negotiations focus on the values of "goods" to be forgone and the values of "goods" to be rewarded. Negotiations in nursing involve many different outcomes, ranging from a one-time action of turning in bed to stopping cigarette smoking, or to other major lifestyle changes. In negotiations, tradeoffs are often made among valued objects by the participants in an effort to arrive at an agreement. A personal value-structure will influence the way tradeoffs are made in negotiations.

*5. Personality explanation.*   Successful negotiations may be attained more often when compatible personalities are negotiating in nurse-client relationships. Other personal characteristics such as affective orientation, independence, and locus of control may also influence negotiations in nursing.

*6. Influence of behavioral skills used in negotiation.*   Nurses who have a broad behavioral repertoire, effective in interaction and exchange, may be more successful in nurse-client negotiations.

*7. Process explanation.*   Negotiations may be studied in terms of ongoing process in a phenomenological sense. The symbolic interactionists' approach in the explanation as to what occurs in the nurse-client negotiation will force us to examine negotiation as a special case in social interaction.

## THE CONCEPT OF NURSING PRACTICE

### Definition

In ordinary nursing terminology, *nursing practice* refers to many different things and is often used interchangeably with "nursing skills," "clinical practice," or simply "nursing." Most often it is used, in a comparative sense, on a par with nursing theory and nursing research. Nursing as a discipline is viewed as having three structural components in this usage: theory, practice, and research.

In a generic sense, practice is considered as the concrete action that is carried out by individuals in a specified situation. The term is used differently from that common usage of "practice," as in "You will improve with practice," in which it is synonymous with "drill." A theoretical conceptualization of practice as used in nursing practice or professional practice is closely linked with another common usage, as in "Your idea is a good one, but it won't work in practice."

Practice as a phenomenon is different from action: (a) Practice presupposes the presence of a mental image of what will be or need be enacted, that is, a mental picture, a cognitive understanding, or knowledge is antecedent to action; and (b) practice is situation-specific. In this light, Agyris and Schon (1976) define professional practice as a sequence of actions undertaken by a person to serve others who are considered clients.

In proposing situation-producing theory as the proper form of nursing theory, Dickoff and James (1975) implicitly equate practice with activities that "produce situation." To them, practice is the vehicle by which a desired situation in nursing is produced, and is theoretically influenced by goal-content, prescription, and a survey list. Theoretically, a survey list infers situational variables relative to prescribed nursing activity. In turn, they also conceive that practice, the activity performed in reality, is the base for descriptive theories (factor-isolating theories) as well.

In a similar point of view, Wilson (1977) proposes that the grounded theory approach proposed by Glaser and Strauss (1967) be adopted to develop theories that are applicable to explaining and predicting processes of nursing practice. Beckstrand (1978a and 1978b) also defines practice as a class of phenomena that includes all actions that bring about changes in an entity for a realization of a greater good.

There is a general agreement on the definition of nursing practice as a theoretical construct. Nursing practice is a set of actions enacted by a nurse (the actor) toward the good of the client in specific situations. The concept involves: (a) knowledge of how to arrive at "good" outcomes of nursing, (b) knowledge of what is "good" for the client, and (c) performance of prescribed nursing actions in reality. The goal of action is always directed toward the client, while the actions in nursing practice are always referrable to the nurse as the originator of "provisions" for the client. The actions in nursing practice are special types of human enactments performed in the context of the service requirements of a client. Practice exists in a given nursing situation as a discrete care apart from all other cases, and is primarily oriented to the values that define what is normatively good for the client.

## Operationalization

Nursing practice refers to the contents of nursing care and is enumerable in a descriptive fashion. The most commonly used variable term for nursing practice is *quality of care*. Quality of nursing care is determined by the nature of nursing actions performed in nursing situations and their effects on the client. Operationalization of nursing practice poses a problem in relation to units of analysis. Definitions and conceptualizations in the nursing literature, so far, have not specified the meanings of practice in terms of spatio-temporal frameworks.

By definition, nursing practice may refer to the phenomena of the nursing profession, the phenomena that exist with the individual nurse in everyday practice in general, or the phenomena of specific action performed by a nurse in a given specific situation. Nursing practice can also be specified according to the type of nursing action, such as in nursing practice of communication or nursing practice of preoperative teaching. It also may be categorized according to client characteristics, such as nursing practice for children, nursing practice for healthy adults, etc. It appears that operationalization of nursing practice has to be made according to the conceptual boundary that is specified in the definition and study.

## Relationships with Other Concepts

The main questions that require scientific explanations regarding the phenomena of nursing practice are: Is it a "good" practice? When is it a "good" practice? To what degree is there a fidelity of implementation in nursing practice with theoretical knowledge? And, what are the effects on practice of those factors exogenous to a scientific, theoretical base?

Although Beckstrand (1978a and 1978b) argues that there is no need for a specific nursing practice theory to answer such questions, it is proposed here that nursing practice theories are necessary to address these questions to the extent that scientific, theoretical knowledge is uniquely assembled for nursing practice and that the contexts of nursing practice are unique from other practice disciplines. Collins and Fielder's arguments for the need for practice theory also seem valid (1981).

By putting such questions more systematically, the following problems emerge, requiring scientific explanations within nursing practice theory framework:

*1. Nursing practice of good quality as influenced by the nature of scientific and theoretical knowledge.* Quality of nursing practice is essentially dependent upon the richness and rigor of scientific knowledge from which the prescriptions of nursing activities are derived. Practice without a scientific foundation will flounder as a result of the inadequacy of trial-and-error by itself.

**2. *Fidelity of implementation.*** The fact that nursing practitioners are educated to use systematic knowledge for practice, and that nursing practice is based on a situation-producing theory, is no guarantee that nursing practice in reality will be implemented accordingly. The issue is how nursing knowledge that is internalized and learned by an individual nurse as a system of individualized knowledge becomes transformed into nursing actions, that is, into knowledge-in-use. What prompts the nurse to behave in a specific way? Is there a mental or psychological explanation that specifies why one nurse might behave differently from another in a given nursing situation, provided that there is a standardized level of knowledge? A nurse's perception of the world and situation, value-structures used to evaluate the situation, personal relationships, psychomotor and cognitive skills of generalized and specialized types that are acquired from experience, and the ability to focus have all been found to influence the degree of congruency between the knowledge and knowledge-use in practice.

**3. *Exogenous influences.*** The atmosphere of practice and its meanings to the nurse, contextual changes that occur within the nursing situation, and the complexity of a situation that requires complicated management of skills are some of the external forces that may influence the nature of nursing practice and nursing-practice outcomes.

Thus, theories of nursing practice should be concerned with these kinds of theoretical and empirical problems. The aim of such theories would be to produce "better" nursing practice, given the scientific knowledge and the constraints of a practice situation.


## SUMMARY

The main idea for this chapter has been to bring about a closure to a circle for conceptualizing nursing phenomena. Nursing action is the core of nursing knowledge and should be understood within the theoretical frameworks of nursing theories. My contention throughout the chapter has been to offer a systematic framework for conceptualizing nursing action phenomena. Once different phenomena are classified into like categories, it becomes clear to theoretical thinkers that discovering and developing theories for nursing phenomena can be pursued in a systematic fashion.

Nursing's theoretical development up until now has paid more attention to developing models to understand phenomena in the domain of client. As shown in this chapter, conceptualization of nursing action in both the client-nurse system and the nurse system are descriptive at best. Theoretical linkages for situation-producing theories must be developed. We also are still struggling with boundary-defining tasks. Subject matter for nursing study and definitions of nursing phenomena can only result from rigorous conceptual and theoretical specifications of the domain of nursing action.

## BIBLIOGRAPHY

Argyris, C, and Schon, DA. *Theory in Practice: Increasing Professional Effectiveness.* San Francisco: Jossey-Bass, 1976

Argyris, C, and Schon, DA. Evaluating Theories of Action. In WG Bennis, KD Nenne, R Chin, and KE Corey (eds.): *The Planning of Change,* Third edition. New York: Holt, Rinehart, and Winston, 1976, pp 137–147

Avant, K. Nursing Diagnosis: Maternal Attachment. *Adv Nurs Sci* 2, no. 1: 45–55, 1979

Beckstrand, J. The Notion of a Practice Theory and the Relationships of Scientific and Ethical Knowledge to Practice. *Res Nurs Health* 1: 131–136, 1978a

Beckstrand, J. The Need for a Practice Theory as Indicated by the Knowledge Used in the Conduct of Practice. *Res Nurs Health* 1: 175–179, 1978b

Beckstrand, J. A Critique of Several Conceptions of Practice Theory in Nursing. *Res Nurs Health* 3: 69–79, 1980

Benne, KD, Chin, R, and Bennis, WG. Science and Practice. In WG Bennis, KD Benne, R Chin, and KE Corey (eds.): *The Planning of Change,* Third edition. New York: Holt, Rinehart, and Winston, 1976, pp 128–137

Blake, M. The Peplau Developmental Model for Nursing Practice. In JP Riehl and SC Roy (eds.): *Conceptual Models for Nursing Practice,* Second edition. New York: Appleton-Century-Crofts, 1980, pp 53–59

Bloch, D. Some Crucial Terms in Nursing: What Do They Really Mean? *Nurs Outlook* 22: 689–694, 1974

Bourdieu, P. *Outline of a Theory of Practice.* Cambridge: Cambridge University Press, 1977

Calley, JM, Dirsen, M, Engalla, M, and Hennrich, ML. The Orem Self-Care Nursing Model. In JP Riehl and SC Roy (eds.): *Conceptual Models for Nursing Practice,* Second edition. New York: Appleton-Century-Crofts, 1980, pp 302–314

Coddington, A. *Theories of the Bargaining Process.* Chicago: Aldine, 1968

Coleman, LJ. Orem's Self-Care Concept of Nursing. In JP Riehl and SC Roy (eds.): *Conceptual Models for Nursing Practice,* Second edition. New York: Appleton-Century-Crofts, 1980, pp 315–328

Collins, RJ, and Fielder, JH. Beckstrand's Concept of Practice Theory: A Critique. *Res Nurs Health* 4: 317–321, 1981

Coser, RL. *Training in Ambiguity.* New York: The Free Press, 1979

Donaldson, SK, and Crowley, DM. The Discipline of Nursing. *Nurs Outlook* 26: 113–120, 1978

Fox, RC. Training for Uncertainty. In RK Merton, GG Reeder, and PL Kendall (eds.): *The Student Physician.* Cambridge, MA: Harvard University Press, 1957

Freidson, E. *Profession of Medicine.* New York: Dodd, Mead, 1970a

Freidson, E. *Professional Dominance.* New York: Atherton Press, 1970b.

Gebbie, KM, and Lavin, MA. *Proceedings of the First National Conference: Classification of Nursing Diagnoses.* St. Louis: C.V. Mosby, 1975

Gordon, M, and Sweeney, MA. Methodological Problems and Issues in Identifying and Standardizing Nursing Diagnosis. *Adv Nurs Sci* 2, no. 1: 1–15, 1979

Graves, C, Katz, J, Nishiyama, Y, Soames, S, Stecher, R, and Tovey, P. Tacit Knowledge. *J Philos* 70: 318–331, 1973

Hall, L. Another View of Nursing Care and Quality. In KM Straub and KS Parker (eds.): *Continuity of Patient Care: The Role of Nursing.* Washington, DC: Catholic University Press, 1966, pp 47–66

Havelock, RG, and Benne, KD. An Exploratory Study of Knowledge Utilization. In WG Bennis, KD Benne, R Chin, and KE Corey (eds.): *The Planning of Change,* Third edition. New York: Holt, Rinehart, and Winston, 1976, pp 151–164

Henderson, B. Nursing Diagnosis: Theory and Practice. *Adv Nurs Sci* 1, no.1: 75–83, 1978

Johnson, DE. *The Behavioral System Model for Nursing.* A Paper Presented at the University of Delaware. Newark, Delaware, 1977

Johnson, DE. The Behavioral System Model for Nursing. In JP Riehl and SC Roy (eds.): *Conceptual Models for Nursing Practice,* Second edition. New York: Appleton-Century-Crofts, 1980, pp 207–216

Jones, PE. A Terminology for Nursing Diagnoses. *Adv Nurs Sci* 2, no. 1: 65–72, 1979

Kim, MJ, and Moritz, DA (eds.). *Classification of Nursing Diagnoses: Proceedings of the Third and Fourth National Conferences.* New York: McGraw-Hill, 1982

King, IM. *Toward a Theory for Nursing.* New York: John Wiley, 1971

King, IM. The Health Care System: Nursing Intervention Subsystem. In H Werley, et al. (eds.): *Health Research: The Systems Approach.* New York: Springer, 1976

King, IM. *A Theory for Nursing: Systems, Concepts, Process.* New York: John Wiley, 1981

Kritek, P. The Generation and Classification of Nursing Diagnoses: Toward a Theory of Nursing. *Image* 10: 33–40, 1978

Kritek, P. Commentary: The Development of Nursing Diagnosis and Theory. *Adv Nurs Sci* 2, no.1: 73–79, 1979

Levine, ME. *Introduction to Clinical Nursing,* Second edition. Philadelphia: F.A. Davis, 1973

McCall, G, and Simmons J. *Identities and Interactions,* Revised edition. New York: The Free Press, 1978

Merton, RK. *Sociological Ambivalence and Other Essays.* New York: The Free Press, 1976

Mundinger, MO, and Jauron, GD. Developing a Nursing Diagnosis. *Nurs Outlook* 23: 94–98, 1975

Neuman, B. The Betty Neuman Health Care Systems Model: A Total Person Approach to Patient Problems. In JP Riehl and SC Roy (eds.): *Conceptual Models for Nursing Practice*, Second edition. New York: Appleton-Century-Crofts, 1980, pp 119–134

Newman, MA. *Theory Development in Nursing*. Philadelphia: F.A. Davis, 1979

The Nursing Theories Conference Group. *Nursing Theories: The Base for Professional Nursing Practice*. Englewood Cliffs, NJ: Prentice-Hall, 1980

Orem, DE. *Nursing: Concepts of Practice*, Second edition. New York: McGraw-Hill, 1980

Orlando, IJ. *The Dynamic Nurse-Patient Relationship: Function, Process, and Principle*. New York: G. Putnam's Sons, 1961

Peplau, HE. *Interpersonal Relations in Nursing*. New York: G. Putnam's Sons, 1962

Peplau, HE. Professional Closeness. *Nurs Forum* 8: 346, 1969

Riehl, JP. The Riehl Interaction Model. In JP Riehl and SC Roy (eds.): *Conceptual Models for Nursing Practice*, Second edition. New York: Appleton-Century-Crofts, 1980, pp 350–356

Riehl, JP, and Roy, SC (eds.). *Conceptual Models for Nursing Practice*, Second edition. New York: Appleton-Century-Crofts, 1980

Rogers, ME. *An Introduction to the Theoretical Basis of Nursing*. Philadelphia: F.A. Davis, 1970

Rogers, ME. Nursing: A Science of Unitary Man. In JP Riehl and SC Roy (eds.): *Conceptual Models for Nursing Practice*, Second edition. New York: Appleton-Century-Crofts, 1980, pp 329–337

Roy SC. A Diagnostic Classification System for Nursing. *Nurs Outlook* 23: 90–94, 1975

Roy, SC. The Roy Adaptation Model. In JP Riehl and SC Roy (eds.): *Conceptual Models for Nursing Practice*, Second edition. New York: Appleton-Century-Crofts, 1980, pp 179–188

Roy, SC, and Roberts, SL. *Theory Construction in Nursing: An Adaptation Model*. Englewood Cliffs, NJ: Prentice-Hall, 1981

Strauss, A. *Negotiations: Varieties, Contexts, Processes, and Social Order*. San Francisco: Jossey-Bass, 1978

Swain, MA, and Steckel, SB. Influencing Adherence among Hypertensives. *Res Nurs Health* 4: 213–222, 1981

von Wright, GH. On So-Called Practical Inference. *Acta Sociologica* 15: 39–54, 1972

Watson, J. *Nursing: The Philosophy and Science of Caring*. Boston: Little, Brown, 1979

Wiedenback, E. *Clinical Nursing: A Helping Art*. New York: Springer, 1964

White, R. Motivation Reconsidered: The Concept of Competence. *Psychol Rev* 66: 297–334, 1956

Young, O (ed.). *Bargaining*. Urbana, IL: University of Illinois Press, 1976

Zartman, IW (ed.). *The Fifty Percent Solution*. Garden City, NY: Doubleday, 1976

# 7

# Development of Theoretical Statements in Nursing

Theories are the key to the scientific understanding of empirical phenomena, and they are normally developed only when previous research has yielded a body of information, including empirical generalizations about the phenomena in question. A theory is then intended to provide deeper understanding by presenting those phenomena as manifestations of certain underlying processes, governed by characteristic laws which account for, and usually correct and refine, the previously established generalizations.

*Carl G. Hempel*

## OVERVIEW

This chapter aims to show the nature of theoretical statement in nursing theories through a careful analysis of currently existing or already developed statements. While the previous chapters are more critically concerned with the nature of concepts within each domain, this chapter is concerned with the nature of theories as they culminate from relevant concepts. Attempts are made to show how concepts delineated within the three domains can be developed into systems of theoretical statements. Here the purpose is not to propose theories, but rather to show what happens to an array of discrete theoretical constructs when they are put into theoretical statements. The idea is to lead to thinking about developing a theoretical system through a systematic and logical linking of concepts that compose nursing's relevance structure.

The chapter presents the types of theoretical statements that deal with nursing phenomena, as they are expressed in the current nursing literature.[1] The purpose is to show how rigorously and with what specificity theoretical statements are expressed and studied in nursing. In addition, the review also indicates to us which nursing phenomena are currently of interest to nursing researchers.

Theoretical statements linking concepts and phenomena within each domain and across the domains are examined in order to indicate that relevant and critical relationships may be brought together in "Theories in Nursing" and "Theories of Nursing." First, we examine the theoretical statements for the domains of client, environment, and nursing action separately; then we proceed to analyze those theoretical systems that deal with theoretical statements that bridge concepts across two or three domains at the same time.

In Chapter 2, the major terms of importance in theory development were defined. A theoretical statement refers to a proposition that links two or more concepts in basically two relational forms: associational relationship, i.e., covariance, and causal relationship. This means that a theoretical statement specifies the relationship of one class of phenomena to another class of phenomena. In this chapter, primarily this definition is used to illustrate the types of theoretical statements examined for our purpose.

## THEORETICAL STATEMENTS AMONG CONCEPTS WITHIN THE DOMAINS

Theoretical statements of concepts referring to phenomena within the same domain are important for two reasons: (a) a set of such theoretical statements may make up a theory for the domain; and (b) such statements lead us to a more refined conceptual system by which phenomena may be reclassified. My approach, consisting of holistic and particularistic conceptualizations of phenomena within domains, also suggests three levels of relationships:

1. a holistic concept with another holistic concept;
2. a holistic concept with a particularistic concept;
3. a particularistic concept with another particularistic concept.

## THE DOMAIN OF CLIENT

In Chapter 4, several conceptualizations regarding phenomena in this domain are presented. Such conceptualizations appear to be related to theoretical models, and were, in most instances, developed in a deductive fashion. On the other hand, the use of the inductive method and a combined inductive and deductive method for conceptual clarification were evident in nursing research literature. Activities related to developing factor-isolating theories were prevalent in the literature reviewed, especially for this domain.

As presented in Table 9, 51 articles (more articles than concepts named in the table, because of duplications) deal with conceptual clarification. This number comprises 16 percent of the total number of articles reviewed for this study (a total number of 316 articles). An additional 17 articles, as shown in Figure 5, deal with relationships between phenomena within the domain of client.

This review shows the kinds of scholarly attention bestowed in nursing studies of client phenomena. These examples also indicate the extensiveness of

**TABLE 9. Concepts and Phenomena Examined in the Published Works in the Selected Nursing Journals\* (1978–1981)—The Domain of Client**

| Holistic | Particularistic |
|---|---|
| Adaptation | Anxiety |
| Adaptation as "healthy" | Attachment behavior |
| Behavioral system | Boredom and confusion |
| Denver developmental system | Child abuse and neglect |
| Depleted health potential | Cognitive development |
| Duration experience | Decision-making |
| Family growth and development | Exploratory behavior |
| Growth vs persistence | Fatigue |
| Health | Fear |
| Health need | Grief |
| Holistic health | Health-belief |
| Independence | Interpersonal conflict in |
| Life event | marital partners |
| Perceived uncertainty in illness | In vitro fertilization |
| Process of recovery | Locus of control |
| Pronominalization | Love |
| Self-care agency | Maternal attachment |
| Stress and coping | Menopause |
| | Neonatal perception |
| | Obesity |
| | Pain |
| | Paternal attachment |
| | Privacy |
| | Psychophysiological |
| | stress |
| | Self-esteem |

\*Nursing journals reviewed for this table are: *Nursing Research, Research in Nursing and Health,* and *Advances in Nursing Science.*

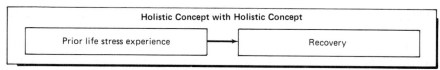

**Holistic Concept with Holistic Concept**

| | |
|---|---|
| Prior life stress experience | → Recovery |

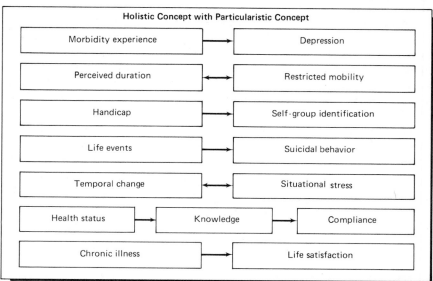

**Holistic Concept with Particularistic Concept**

| | |
|---|---|
| Morbidity experience | → Depression |
| Perceived duration | ↔ Restricted mobility |
| Handicap | → Self-group identification |
| Life events | → Suicidal behavior |
| Temporal change | ↔ Situational stress |
| Health status | → Knowledge → Compliance |
| Chronic illness | → Life satisfaction |

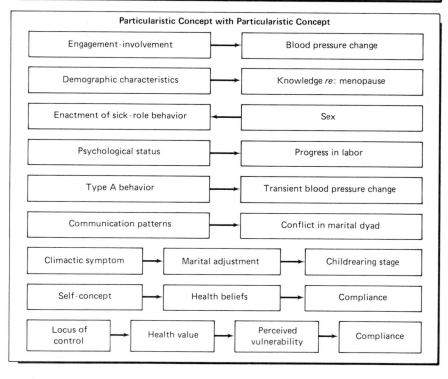

**Particularistic Concept with Particularistic Concept**

| | |
|---|---|
| Engagement-involvement | → Blood pressure change |
| Demographic characteristics | → Knowledge *re*: menopause |
| Enactment of sick-role behavior | ← Sex |
| Psychological status | → Progress in labor |
| Type A behavior | → Transient blood pressure change |
| Communication patterns | → Conflict in marital dyad |
| Climactic symptom | → Marital adjustment → Childrearing stage |
| Self-concept | → Health beliefs → Compliance |
| Locus of control | → Health value → Perceived vulnerability → Compliance |

subject matter that has been selected as appropriate nursing concerns. The concepts studied at this stage (descriptive) are somewhat different from those studied in propositional forms as shown in Figure 5. More abstract concepts are studied on the conceptual-clarification level as compared to the propositional-level studies. Examples from Figure 5 show that theoretical statements relating one particularistic concept to another particularistic concept are more commonly tested. The conceptual foci of particularistic phenomena vary from physiological phenomena (e.g., blood pressure change) to highly perceptual phenomena (e.g., perceived vulnerability).

While these indicate as examples the kinds of theoretical statements being examined in research and/or conceptual studies, the major theoretical statements are found in the theoretical models that have been developed in nursing. In the next section, an examination is made of the theoretical statements specified in the nursing theoretical models by Rogers, Roy, Orem, and King, excerpting from these selected theorists' works that have been discussed in the previous chapters. This examination takes a critical look at the extent to which the existing nursing models are appropriate for empirical studies, and the degree of deductive applications in the empirical studies.

### Rogers' Unitary Man

*1. Man is a unified whole possessing his own integrity and manifesting characteristics that are more than and different from the sum of his parts (1980, p. 47).*   In this proposition, a person is a concept possessing variable characteristics that are compared to another concept, the sum of the person's parts. The proposition is a comparative, rather than a relational one.

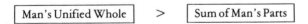

*2. Self-regulation in man is directed toward achieving increasing complexity of organization in man (1970, p. 64).*   Here, one holistic concept of self-regulation is related to another holistic concept of complexity of organization.

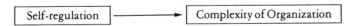

*3. Man's capacity for experiencing himself and his world identifies his humanness (1970, p. 73).*   The concept of capacity, which may be expressed in quantitative and/or qualitative terms, is related to a qualitative concept of "humanness." By capacity for experiencing oneself, Rogers means capacity for creative

*Figure 5.* Relationships between concepts within the domain of client as evidenced in the published works in the selected nursing journals (1978–1981).

potential and sentience. The capacity for experiencing is a process concept of a holistic type, while humanness is a property concept of a holistic nature.

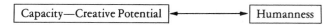

Several other propositions in Rogers' model deal with concepts within the domain of client. It is evident that Rogers' model encompasses theoretical statements that connect holistic phenomena in the domain of client. This suggests that units of analysis for these propositions in Rogers' model must be holistic in nature and refer to phenomena in the client as a whole. In addition, Rogers' model contains three major propositions that deal with concepts in the domain of client and in the domain of environment, which are discussed in a later section.

### Roy Adaptation Model

Roy and Roberts (1981) present a set of nine propositions relating to the regulator subsystem phenomena and another set of twelve propositions relating to the cognator subsystem phenomena as the basic propositions for the theory of the person as an adaptive system. Although their original propositions are intended for explanations of particularistic phenomena conceptually located in each of the subsystems, the following three generalized propositions have been derived from them at a higher level of abstraction. I believe that it is possible to categorize these two sets of 21 propositions into the three groups of the generalized type.

*1. Stimuli proposition: Characteristics of internal and external stimuli a person receives influence his or her adaptive responses.*    Although stimuli may originate in the person's external environment, the concept of stimuli to Roy centers on their characteristics as they are put into the system, and the variabilities in the stimuli's characteristics are not absolute, but relative to the preceding adaptation level. Therefore, this proposition relates the "interpreted" characteristics of stimuli to responses that occur by various processing mechanisms.

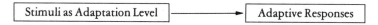

*2. Integrity Proposition: Structural and functional integrities of subsystems of a person influence his or her adaptive responses.*    This proposition relates the system-states with respect to structure and functioning and adaptive responses of the person. It suggests that the kinds of adaptive responses exhibited by an individual are influenced by the level of structural and functional integrity that a subsystem has.

Structural and Functional Integrity ─────▶ Adaptive Responses

*3. Mastery Proposition: Mastery with which a person responds to stimuli influ-ences consequent processing of internal and external stimuli.*   This proposition refers to the feedback nature of the adaptation level, relating the past experi-ences with stimuli as influencing future adaptation.

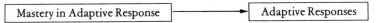

Although the way these three propositions have been summarized appears to indicate that the propositions in the model relate holistic concepts, that is not the case. On the contrary, the majority of the propositions in the theory as stated originally by the authors relate particularistic phenomena to other particularistic phenomena (see Roy and Roberts, 1981). For example, *"increase in short-term or long-term memory will positively influence the effective choice of psycho-motor responses to neural input."*[2] I categorize this proposition as one of the mastery propositions. In this proposition, two particularistic concepts, increase in memory and psychomotor responses to neural input, are related. Roy and Roberts (1981) advanced propositions that pose relationships among particular-istic phenomena in the self-concept, role-function, and interdependence modes of adaptation, as well as those in the physiological needs mode. These also may be categorized into the three general propositions. Roy Adaptation Model also is composed of three major propositions that are concerned with concepts in the domain of client and those in the domain of environment. These propositions are statements that link concepts across the domains and are discussed in the next section.

### Orem's Self-care Model

Of ten propositions that Orem presents within her theory of self-care (Orem, 1980), two propositions specify relationships between concepts within the do-main of client (presented in this section), and two others deal with relationships between phenomena in the domain of client and in the domain of environment. Six propositions are descriptive statements, characterizing the natures of self-care and self-care requisites.

*1. Self-care requisites are partly common to all human beings, but also vary ac-cording to individual's developmental and health states (1980, p. 29).*   The concept of self-care requisite as holistic phenomena in the client is qualitatively related to developmental and health-state variations in the individual.

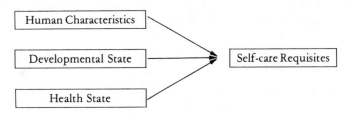

*2. Universal self-care requisites and ways of meeting them may be modified by the age, sex, or developmental or health state of individuals.*   In a similar manner as the first proposition, two holistic concepts, universal self-care requisite and self-care attainment, are related to other human characteristics such as age, sex, developmental state, and health state. This may be, in fact, separated into eight simple propositional statements.

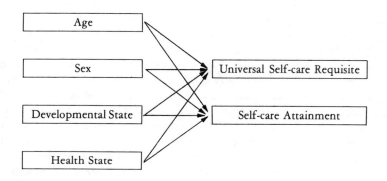

### King's Theory of Goal Attainment
In her theory of goal attainment, King's major emphasis is the interpersonal system. However, she has advanced a few propositions for understanding and explaining phenomena in the personal system.

*1. An individual's perceptions of self, of body image, of time, and space influence the way he or she responds to persons, objects, and events in his or her life (1981, p. 19).*   The proposition relates two concepts: an individual's perceptions and an individual's responses. The concept of an individual's perceptions is delineated to indicate only those perceptions one holds about self and body image that are the aspects of oneself, and about space and time that are aspects of the external world. Even though this concept refers to environment on a secondary level, the focus is not on the actual phenomena of environment themselves, but on how an individual perceives certain aspects of the environment. Therefore, empirically as well as conceptually, such perceptions are the properties of the individual. The dependent variable concept is an individual's responses to persons, objects, and events. King includes action, reaction, and interaction in her conceptualization of human responses.

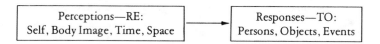

*2. As individuals grow and develop through the life span, experiences with changes in structure and function of their bodies over time influence their perception of self (1981, p. 19).*    Two concepts defining phenomena within an individual, (a) changes in structure and function of body and (b) self-perception, are related in this proposition. This is a less general proposition, compared to the first one.

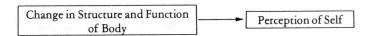

*3. As a person's experiences and perceptions change, his or her body image changes (1981, p. 32).*    These two propositions (Propositions 2 and 3) suggest variability in perceptions of self and body image, which are considered as independent variables in Proposition 1. Here, these concepts have been considered as dependent variables. The concept of perception refers to general perception.

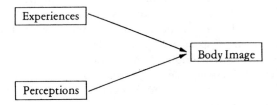

*4. One's perception is related to past experiences, to concept of self, to biological inheritance, to educational background, and to socioeconomic groups (1981, p. 20).*    Contrary to the first proposition, the concept of perception in this proposition refers to "generalized awareness" of reality, and is considered as a dependent variable concept. Selection of the independent variable concepts for this proposition are derived from accepted knowledge in the scientific field.

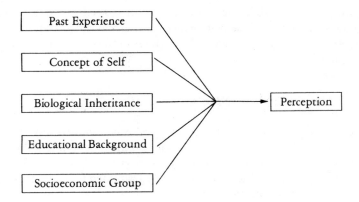

*5. Individual growth and development are [partly] functions of genetic endowment, and meaningful and satisfying experiences (1981, p. 31).* The nature of an individual's growth and development is linked to biological givens and life experiences in this proposition, and the proposition deals with holistic concepts in the domain of client.

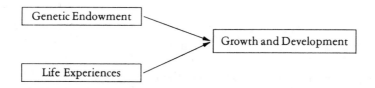

To King, these are the main explanatory characteristics of the personal system as the person is considered by itself. She proposes five main concepts (perception, self, body image, space, and time) in the personal system as major elements describing the human person, and advances propositions specifying factors that influence the phenomena of perception in general, and specific to self and body-image. However, she does not present specific propositions regarding the phenomena of space perception and time perception. There is also a circularity in the conceptualization of "perceptions" as they are treated in the same propositions as "general" and "specific" to certain facets of the human person. Therefore, understanding and explaining the phenomena of the personal system remains incomplete.

These examples of propositions found in the selected theoretical models of nursing suggest that there is need for greater specification of theoretical formulations dealing with phenomena within the domain of client. The primary theoretical problems inherent in these examples are incompleteness and logical inadequacy. They also point up areas for empirical testing of human phenomena from the nursing perspective. These propositions have weak connections with the theoretical statements found in empirical literature, suggesting that nursing studies are heavily using theories from other scientific fields. This suggests a certain readiness and ease with which nursing scientists are applying theories from other fields, and a potential for richness in the development of "theories in nursing."

## THE DOMAIN OF ENVIRONMENT

Phenomena in the domain of environment have been examined very little in the nursing literature. One important reason may be that environmental phenomena *by themselves* are not important subject matter for nursing. Only two concepts, social support and ethical structure, were examined for conceptual clarification in the reviewed nursing literature.

There were neither theoretical nor empirical studies dealing with propositions relating phenomena within the domain of environment alone. However, there were studies and theoretical statements that examined relationships between phenomena in the domain of client and those in the domain of environment. Indeed, it appears that phenomena in the domain of environment are essential for nursing attention to the extent that they are linked to phenomena of either the client or nursing action.

Hence, a generation of theoretical statements linking phenomena within the domain of environment itself may have an insignificant value to nursing science. It may belong to other bodies of knowledge, such as physics, ecology, etc. Nevertheless, there is a need to develop a clearer conceptualization of certain environmental phenomena as they are applied to the problems of nursing proper. The concepts of social support, emotional atmosphere, territory, esthetic environment, noise, etc., need conceptualizations from a nursing perspective if we are to apply such concepts for an understanding of human phenomena of interest to nursing.

## THE DOMAIN OF NURSING ACTION

In Chapter 6, many phenomena of this domain were discussed within several theoretical models. Conceptual clarification is an ongoing process, and is evidenced in the review done on the nursing literature (Table 10). The recent peri-

**TABLE 10. Concepts and Phenomena Examined in the Published Works in the Selected Nursing Journals\* (1978–1981)—The Domain of Nursing Action**

| The Client-Nurse System | The Nurse System |
|---|---|
| Avoidance | Assessment behavior |
| Caring | Charting behavior |
| Empathy | Expert behavior |
| Holistic nursing | Health-risk appraisal |
| Interpersonal complementarity | Moral judgment in |
| Interpersonal value conflict | nursing dilemma |
| Language of touch | Nursing diagnosis |
| Prevention | Nursing documentation |
| Self-instructional model | Nursing judgment |
| in counseling | Pattern of knowing |
| Stress management | Practice theory |
| | Prediction in diagnostic |
| | task |
| | Professional account- |
| | ability |
| | Quality assurance |

\*Nursing journals reviewed for this table are: *Nursing Research, Research in Nursing and Health,* and *Advances in Nursing Science.*

odical literature indicates that there is a greater number of articles examining phenomena of nursing action in the nurse system than in the client-nurse system. It is interesting since the formal theoretical development has focused more on the client-nurse system rather than on the nurse system. A total of 27 articles (9 percent) deal with conceptualization of phenomena in the nursing action domain. An additional eight articles tested relationships between phenomena within the nursing action domain, as shown in Figure 6. Evidence indicates that there are attempts to clarify and conceptualize the meanings and operationalizations of phenomena that have been treated rather carelessly in the past. Empathy, caring, and holistic nursing are examples.

The development of such strategies as stress management, touch, and contracting defined as nursing interventions shows nursing's attempts to expand the repertoire of nursing therapies. Theoretical statements inferrable from the relationships studied for phenomena within the nursing action domain as shown

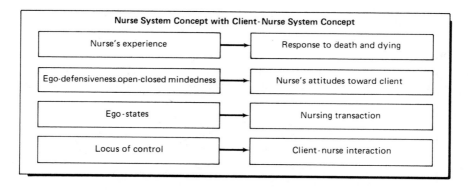

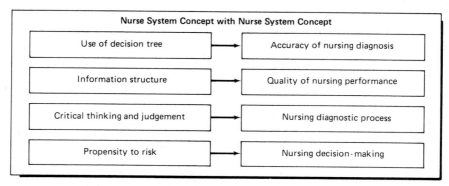

*Figure 6.* Relationships between concepts within the domain of nursing action as evidenced in the published works in the selected nursing journals (1978–1981).

in Figure 6 again confirm my contention that there is a need for development of nursing practice theories that can systematize relationships among phenomena within the domain of nursing action. As evident in these relationships, the loci of nurse system phenomena encompass: (a) trait characteristics of the nurse, (b) experiential phenomena, (c) informational and knowledge structure, (d) attitudes of the nurse, and (e) intellectual and psychomotor skills. The lack of systematic explanations for this area of nursing phenomena should impress upon the nursing scientists the need to make theoretical developments in this area a priority.

There still exists much work to be done to refine our understanding and explanation of phenomena within the domains, especially the client and nursing action domains. A paucity of empirical studies applying nursing theoretical models is also apparent. Prescriptive theories depend upon knowledge generated by descriptive and explanatory theories. Thus, the key to a scientific practice of nursing is in having a more systematic understanding of what is happening with the client and of how we behave in nursing situations.

## THEORETICAL STATEMENTS AMONG CONCEPTS ACROSS THE DOMAINS

In this chapter, I present evidence of theoretical statements generated in published studies to show the kinds of questions that are asked in nursing. An examination is also made of selected propositions presented in the previously discussed theoretical models. My purpose is primarily to show foundations from which more refined theoretical thinking can be generated within the science of nursing.

## THE DOMAIN OF CLIENT AND ENVIRONMENT

The conceptualization of humanity in nursing has usually placed a person within his or her environment. Rarely in nursing do we think of a person without having some relationships with the environment. Explanations of many client phenomena are made in terms of environmental phenomena accordingly.

Figure 7 lists examples of explanations that are found in the current periodical literature. In most of these cases, environmental phenomena are independent variables, indicating that the focus of explanation in nursing studies is the client.

Phenomena of physical environment, such as thermal application, auditory stimulation, and territorial intrusion, as well as the phenomena of social environment, such as social support, are both examined in nursing. Phenomena of symbolic environment, however, are rarely treated in the literature. This may be

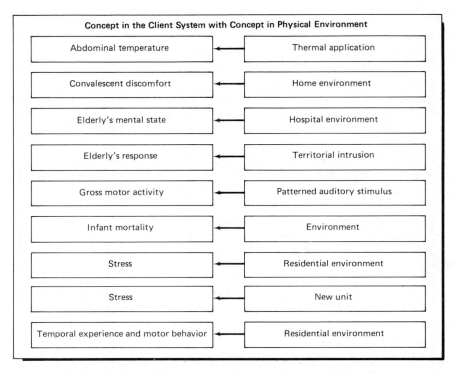

*Figure 7.* Relationships between concept in the domain of client and concept in the domain of environment as evidenced in the published works in the selected nursing journals (1978–1981).

an artifact of the review presented here, which included analysis of only three nursing research journals over the past four years. It is possible that many nursing studies dealing with phenomena of the symbolic environment are present in other journals in sociology and anthropology.

Propositions found in nursing theorists' work relating phenomena in the domain of client to phenomena in the domain of environment are not as comprehensive as those found for explanations with the domain of client.

## Rogers' Unitary Man

*Man-environment transactions are characterized by continuous repatterning of both man and environment. The constant interchange of matter and energy between man and environment is at the basis of human's becoming (1970, pp. 53–54).* Rogers' conceptualization of synergistic repatterning between a person and the environment is expressed in this proposition. This proposition is also based on the assumption that person-environment transactions result in new,

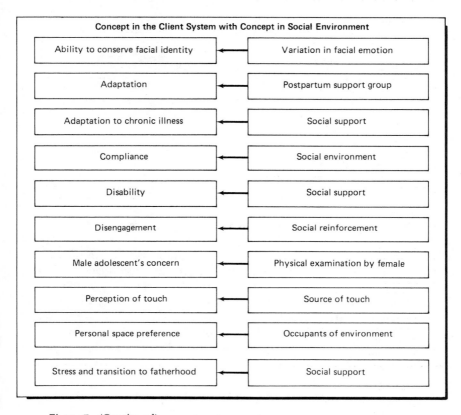

*Figure 7.* (Continued)

evolving, and more complex patterns and organizations of both systems. This proposition is further divided into three ''principles of homeodynamics,'' as follows (1980, p. 333):

1. *Principle of Helicy*

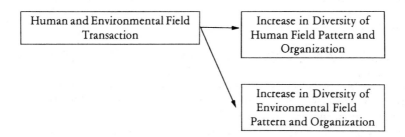

2. *Principle of Resonancy*

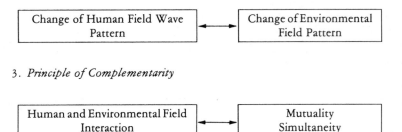

3. *Principle of Complementarity*

These three principles characterize the relationships between the human field and the environmental field. The main weakness in Rogers' principles as theoretical statements can be traced to her basic assumption of evolution and the creativity of life. These are concepts that are based on unidirectionality of change and noncausality. Therefore, these principles are basically oriented to explaining the "speed" with which change (i.e., change in terms of diversity, complexity, and wave-length) occurs in human and environmental fields. Nursing scientists are having some difficulties with operationalizations of the concepts, as well as with bringing the abstractness of the concepts and the relationships to an empirical level for testing.

**Roy Adaptation Model**
Roy's stimuli propositions include the idea of environment, to the extent that part of a given set of stimuli may originate from the person's environment. Phenomena in the domain of environment are significant in the theoretical model insofar as they represent stimuli input to the person.

For this reason, Roy's model does not contain specific propositions that suggest relationships between the client phenomena and the environmental phenomena, as they relate to the mode of physiological needs. However, for the self-concept, role-function, and interdependence modes of adaptation in the model, the stimuli propositions have been specified with respect to phenomena of the environmental domain.

*1. The positive quality of social experience in the form of others' approvals positively influences the level of feelings of adequacy (1981, p. 255).* The proposition deals with particularistic phenomena in the domain of social environment, the approval of others, and particularistic phenomena in the domain of client, feelings of adequacy.

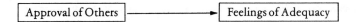

2. *The amount of clarity of input in the form of role cues and cultural norms positively influences the adequacy of role-taking (1981, p. 267).* The proposition relates aspects of symbolic environment to phenomena in the domain of client. Explanation is also on a particularistic level.

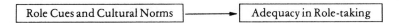

3. *The optimum amount of environmental changes positively influences the adequacy of seeking nurturance and nurturing (1981, p. 277).* The proposition takes the phenomena of environment in a holistic manner and relates a holistic environmental phenomenon, environmental change, to phenomena in the domain of client, the behaviors of seeking nurturance and nurturing.

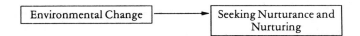

These three propositions deal with phenomena of social environment (approval of others), phenomena of symbolic environment (role cues and cultural norms), and phenomena of the total environment (environmental change). Dependent variables of the propositions are in the domain of client in terms of human perception, behavior, and functioning. One theoretical concern of note with these propositions is the lack of connectedness, i.e., integration between these propositions' explanatory orientations and the general adaptation-level propositions.

### Orem's Self-care Model

Orem advances two propositions that relate human phenomena to environmental factors in the self-care model:

1. *Self-care is learned within the context of social groups by human interaction and communication (1980, p. 28).*

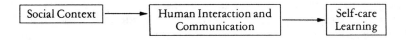

2. *Some self-care requisites have their origins in the environment (1980, p. 29).* The proposition postulates a general relationship between the environment and

the self-care requisite a person will have. In this proposition, Orem conceptualizes environment in a holistic manner. However, the meaning of this proposition is not very clear.

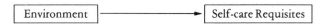

### King's Theory of Goal Attainment

King proposes one proposition relating phenomena of environment and phenomena in the domain of client. Environmental phenomena of interest in the proposition are physical objects and social elements. The dependent variable of concern is a person's growth and development.

*The manner in which a person grows and develops is influenced by other people and objects in the environment (1981, p. 31).*

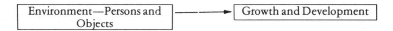

These examples of theoretical statements indicate the extent to which theoretical development in nursing with respect to phenomena in the client and environment exists. Our understanding regarding this area is far from comprehensive. Needless to say, we should raise many more general as well as specific theoretical questions that may lead us to gain an understanding of human phenomena in the environmental contexts. One area of nursing intervention certainly lies in the appropriate control of environmental forces.

The effects of noise on recovery, environmental stimulation on newborn infants' responses, and technology on a person's problem-solving ability are a few of the empirical questions that might be of theoretical interest from the nursing perspective.

## THE DOMAIN OF ENVIRONMENT AND NURSING ACTION

There is only one study in the literature review that dealt with phenomena in these two domains: the relationship between a nurse's informed behavior and nursing culture. This fact may be an artifact also of the review used in this analysis. It is appropriate to assume that phenomena within these two domains are subjects of study in many other fields, such as psychology, sociology, and anthropology. In addition, phenomena of the environment are often considered as intervening or extraneous variables in many studies dealing with phenomena in the client and nursing action domains. Often, phenomena of the environment are included in dynamic relationships, especially in theoretical formulations having a systems perspective. Phenomena of the environment are rarely the primary focus of scientific attention in nursing.

## THE DOMAINS OF CLIENT AND NURSING ACTION

Theoretical statements relating client phenomena and nursing action are oriented toward developing prescriptive theories. There were 41 periodicals (13 percent of the total reviewed) that test relationships between client phenomena and nursing action phenomena, as shown in Figure 8.

Nursing strategies vary from very specific, e.g., positioning, diet, temperature, and prenatal nipple conditioning, to more general nursing interventions, e.g., therapeutic touch, caring, and biofeedback. Client phenomena also vary from very particularistic phenomena, e.g., hypertension, pressure sores, and urinary pH, to holistic phenomena, e.g., distress, self-care, and crisis.

In Roy's model, propositions of nursing prescription are not specified, but are inherent in the premise that nursing treatment follows from nursing diagnosis in which ineffective responses and behaviors are identified as problematic. Since the stimuli are thought to cause behavior, nursing treatment consisting of changing the stimuli can be derived from a nursing diagnosis (Roy and Roberts, 1981). Therefore, specific nursing treatments may be identified for specific ineffective response situations. Yet this theoretical linkage in the model is inferred rather than explicitly stated, except only in terms of manipulation of contextual stimuli. Inferences of the same type are also proposed in Orem's model, in which nursing actions are prescribed in response to the specific level and type of self-care deficit in the client. On the other hand, Rogers' model does not conceptually permit specific propositions that relate the client phenomena to nursing intervention. Nursing interventions are prescribed according to the principles of homeodynamics. Only King proposes a specific set of propositions linking the client phenomena and nursing action phenomena.

### King's Theory of Goal Attainment
King presents a system of eight propositions for a theory of goal attainment in which nursing action phenomena of interaction and transaction are brought together with the client phenomena of goal attainment. The eight propositions are summarized in Figure 9. In a more straightforward manner, this set of propositions may be reduced as follows:

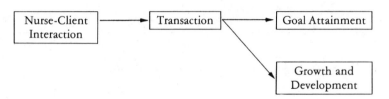

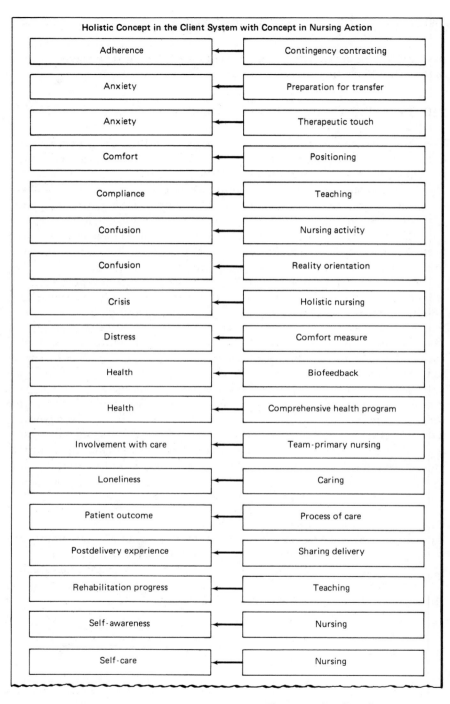

| Holistic Concept in the Client System | with Concept in Nursing Action |
|---|---|
| Adherence | Contingency contracting |
| Anxiety | Preparation for transfer |
| Anxiety | Therapeutic touch |
| Comfort | Positioning |
| Compliance | Teaching |
| Confusion | Nursing activity |
| Confusion | Reality orientation |
| Crisis | Holistic nursing |
| Distress | Comfort measure |
| Health | Biofeedback |
| Health | Comprehensive health program |
| Involvement with care | Team-primary nursing |
| Loneliness | Caring |
| Patient outcome | Process of care |
| Postdelivery experience | Sharing delivery |
| Rehabilitation progress | Teaching |
| Self-awareness | Nursing |
| Self-care | Nursing |

*Figure 8.* (Continued on next page)

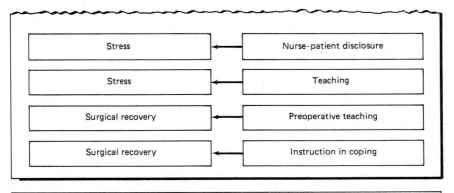

| Stress | ← | Nurse-patient disclosure |
| Stress | ← | Teaching |
| Surgical recovery | ← | Preoperative teaching |
| Surgical recovery | ← | Instruction in coping |

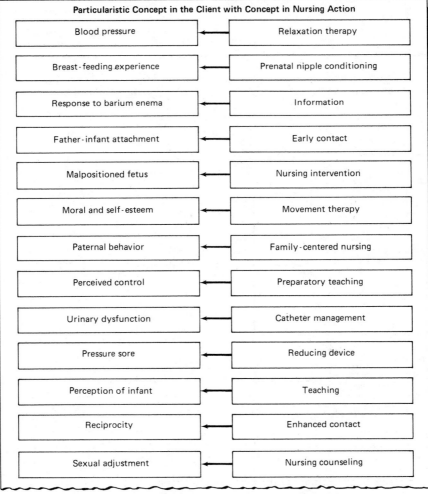

**Particularistic Concept in the Client with Concept in Nursing Action**

| Blood pressure | ← | Relaxation therapy |
| Breast-feeding experience | ← | Prenatal nipple conditioning |
| Response to barium enema | ← | Information |
| Father-infant attachment | ← | Early contact |
| Malpositioned fetus | ← | Nursing intervention |
| Moral and self-esteem | ← | Movement therapy |
| Paternal behavior | ← | Family-centered nursing |
| Perceived control | ← | Preparatory teaching |
| Urinary dysfunction | ← | Catheter management |
| Pressure sore | ← | Reducing device |
| Perception of infant | ← | Teaching |
| Reciprocity | ← | Enhanced contact |
| Sexual adjustment | ← | Nursing counseling |

*Figure 8.* (Continued on next page)

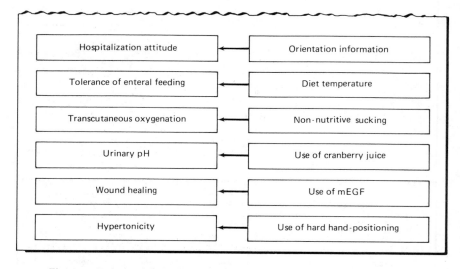

**Figure 8.** Relationship between concepts in the domain of client and concepts in the domain of nursing action as evidenced in the published works in the selected nursing journals (1978–1981).

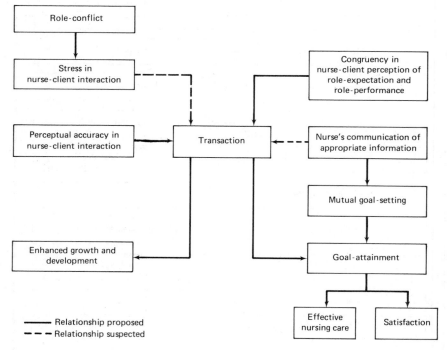

**Figure 9.** Propositions of the theory of goal attainment by King. Adapted from Imogene M. King, *A Theory for Nursing: Systems, Concepts, Processes* (New York: John Wiley, 1981)—Summary of proposed and suspected relationships among the concepts.

Perceptual accuracy, stress, congruency of role perception, role-conflict, and use of communication skills may be included in the concept of nurse-client interaction as elements of variables. In fact, King does this in her discussions of the interpersonal system, and she views communication, transaction, role, and stress as the major variables in the system (King, 1981).

## SUMMARY

This *provisional look* suggests a need to develop systems of theoretical statements dealing with phenomena appropriate for nursing attention at several different levels and with different focuses. Indeed, theoretical questions for the domain of client, environment, and nursing action can be appropriately addressed on three levels of theories: grand theories, middle range theories, and micro theories.

*1. Grand theories.*    The models by Rogers, Roy, and Orem, among others, may be extended to include propositions that link client phenomena of holistic and particularistic types with nursing actions. Grand theories will contain propositions dealing with nursing problems that may exist in various types of clients and nursing-care situations. Thus, grand theories should be comprehensive in their explanations of nursing phenomena. A grand theory of nursing should contain a complex system of propositions, based on assumptions about humanity, health, environment, and nursing action.

*2. Middle range theories.*    King's system of propositions for the theory of goal attainment is an example of a middle range theory. A theory of patient teaching is emerging in the literature, as propositions are being tested with a variety of clients (e.g., surgical patients, pregnant couples, children, hypertensive clients, and the elderly). As a middle range theory, this theory of patient teaching may be applied to explaining and/or influencing such client phenomena as compliance, distress, anxiety, coping, recovery, and rehabilitation.

Theoretical and empirical studies of empathy are also developing into a middle range theory, encompassing such client phenomena as loneliness, withdrawal, depression, pain, dying, and stress. There are many more appropriate areas for development of middle range theories, such as theories of comfort, nurse-client interaction, pain, energy transfer, and collaboration.

*3. Micro theories.*    Many micro-theory developments are in progress. Theoretical efforts dealing with a limited range of application, such as maternal attachment, pressure sores, wound healing, and positioning, have culminated in micro theories. In many instances, as theoretical development becomes enriched, several micro theories together may become a middle range theory. Micro theories provide the backbone for more general, complex theories. Efforts in micro-theory development are also closely related to efforts in empirical generalization, which some scientists value as the first step in theory development.

Our efforts in theoretical developments should be continued on all three levels if we are to develop a knowledge system that offers comprehensive "answers" to nursing questions that are posed for different domains.

My "casualness" in the review of the periodical literature presented in this chapter should not hamper the usefulness of the analysis presented here. The examples shown in this chapter are indeed only examples of (a) what might be appropriate to question for nursing study, (b) what might be necessary for explanations, and (c) how phenomena might be approached for different kinds of explanations. The nursing perspective, the nursing way of viewing the "reality," comes out more clearly in these examples, even if the examples are from a biased sample. By no means are the examples noted in this chapter intended to be taken as representative or comprehensive. Yet they tell the story about the status of nursing in terms of subject matter and theoretical concerns. The burden, then, is on the systematic thinkers, who must strive to define, classify, codify, and explain whatever is essential for what we are all about, *nursing*.

## BIBLIOGRAPHY

Hempel, CG. *Fundamentals of Concept Formation in Empirical Science.* Chicago: University of Chicago Press, 1952

Kaplan, A. *The Conduct of Inquiry: Methodology for Behavioral Science.* San Francisco: Chandler Publishing Company, 1964

King, IM. *A Theory for Nursing: Systems, Concepts, Process.* New York: John Wiley, 1981

The Nursing Theories Conference Group. *Nursing Theories: The Base for Professional Nursing Practice.* Englewood Cliffs, NJ: Prentice-Hall, 1980

Orem, DE. *Nursing: Concepts of Practice,* Second edition. New York: McGraw-Hill, 1980

Riehl, JP, and Roy, SC (eds.). *Conceptual Models for Nursing Practice,* Second edition. New York: Appleton-Century-Crofts, 1980

Rogers, ME. *An Introduction to the Theoretical Basis of Nursing.* Philadelphia: F.A. Davis, 1970

Rogers, ME. Nursing: A Science of Unitary Man. In JP Riehl and SC Roy (eds.): *Conceptual Models for Nursing Practice,* Second edition. New York: Appleton-Century-Crofts, 1980, pp 329–337

Roy, SC. The Roy Adaptation Model. In JP Riehl and SC Roy (eds.): *Conceptual Models for Nursing Practice,* Second edition. New York: Appleton-Century-Crofts, 1980, pp 179–188

Roy, SC, and Roberts, SL. *Theory Construction in Nursing: An Adaptation Model.* Englewood Cliffs, NJ: Prentice-Hall, 1981

# 8

# Concluding Remarks: Issues in Theoretical Development in Nursing

> There must be a clear and distinct separation of the subjective and objective components in any situation in order for us to take rational hold of the problem. The objective problem, thus isolated, is to be dealt with by a logical procedure that seeks to resolve it into a finite number of steps or operations.
>
> *William Barrett*

The discipline of nursing has been subjected to some grand and also to some stifling effects of modern developments and philosophies within the scientific world. By arriving late at the scene of twentieth-century scientific development, nursing's scientific movement, in a way, had to adopt quickly the prevailing ideas of how scientific theories should be developed and what structure theories should have. Nursing science had to adopt behaviors similar to those adopted by developing countries in their efforts to "catch up" with the accomplishments of the developed countries. Nursing had to scramble, leap, and make far-reaching connections in order to catch up with the developments taking place in many scientific fields. Now, we are at a stage where our development of scientific knowledge has to go beyond "what nursing is all about" to "what problems nursing knowledge can 'take on' as its subject matter."

The discipline has approached development of scientific knowledge in a multifaceted fashion. On the one hand, the prevailing attitudes of logical positivism have encouraged and stimulated a few scientists in nursing to follow the route of empirical generalizations. However, because there has been so little systematically presented empirical evidence in nursing, theories based on inductive generalizations have not been well developed. Isolated cases of empirical generalizations have not reached the level of inductive hypotheses (either deterministic or probabilistic) that are required for development of theories. Lately, nursing scientists have rediscovered this inductive method of generating knowledge, especially adopting the position taken by Glaser and Strauss for "discovering grounded theories."

On the other hand, several other nursing theorists and researchers have been engaged in theory development in the spirit of Toulmin. Toulmin (1967 and 1972) suggests that the function of science is to build up systems of explanatory techniques and that theories in science are devices used to describe and explain phenomena in a scientific field. To Toulmin, it is proper or even preferable in science to introduce "theories, techniques of representation, and terminologies together, at one swoop" (1953, p. 146). Toulmin further suggests that scientific problems facing a discipline at a given time are posed by the differences between the intellectual explanatory ideals of a discipline and its current capacity to account for the phenomena in the scientific domain (1972).

Nursing scientists, in general, appear to be following this position for scientific development in nursing. Thus, the maturity of a scientific discipline is present in the way rational objectivity is adopted by the scientific community to select and maintain those conceptual schemes that have a relatively higher ability to resolve the conceptual problems of the discipline.

Through the use of deductive logic, theory development is also possible, although there is no evidence that any nursing scientist is seriously committed to this method.

The discipline of nursing is experiencing an influx of many types and levels of understanding regarding the problems of the discipline. It may be useful, thus, to file a "status report" regarding scientific advancement. My summarization of this status report deals with (a) identification of subject matter, (b) conceptual clarification, (c) nursing orientations or philosophies, (d) theory development, (e) methodology, and (f) the theory-practice-research link.

## IDENTIFICATION OF SUBJECT MATTER

Donaldson and Crowley (1978) summarized three themes that recur in the literature as the essence of nursing: (a) concern with principles and laws that govern the life processes, well-being, and optimum functioning of a human being—sick or well; (b) concern with the patterning of human behavior in interaction with the environment in critical life situations; and (c) concern with the processes by which positive changes in health status are affected. These three themes agree with the domains of client, environment, and nursing action proposed in this book as the fundamental categorization scheme for phenomena essential for nursing studies.

Fawcett (1979) also categorizes essential phenomena in nursing theory as man, health, environment, and nursing. While there is a general agreement in the typology of nursing's subject matter, the actual delineation of subject matter within the typology is still tentative. The evidence has been presented in Chapters 6 and 7. The basic premise for our attempts has to be that of elasticity in identifying disciplinary boundaries.

Identifying subject matter for nursing has to come about within the nursing discipline. This, I believe, can be accomplished by taking a nursing perspective for conceiving of and analyzing phenomena in the three domains. Pain as a phenomenon, for example, can be made an appropriate subject matter for nursing by conceptualizing it from a specific nursing perspective that is different from a medical, biological, or psychological perspective. Therefore, identification of subject matter is a definitional issue that has to be performed with a clear idea of what the nursing perspective consists of.

## CONCEPTUAL CLARIFICATION

Activities in conceptual clarification are the first-level scientific work that culminates in theories. This phase of theoretical work is especially important when a scientific discipline is striving to develop theories and theoretical systems, transplanting many concepts that have been developed in other scientific fields. Conceptual clarification requires analytic and empirical identification of definitional terms.

A concept is selected as appropriate subject matter for a scientific explanation from the nursing perspective; the level of abstraction for conceptual analysis becomes defined; definitional terms for the concept are organized into an interlinked system in order to have a theoretically appropriate meaning; empirical referents are identified; empirical inquiry is made of the definitional meanings; and the definitional terms are reaffirmed, refined, and revised. These are phases for conceptual clarification. Currently, conceptual clarification that is fervently pursued in nursing for the concept of empathy is an example of pretheoretical work that points toward development of a theory.

Conceptual clarification may also serve to redefine, narrow, or broaden concepts that have already been used in theoretical systems. By combining both inductive and deductive methods in the process, concepts become more clearly and rigorously defined and differentiated from similar concepts.

## NURSING ORIENTATIONS OR PHILOSOPHIES

Orientations and philosophies regarding nursing influence the way nursing's subject matter is viewed, and provide the general frameworks within which theories and research methodologies are developed in nursing.

The general world views of nursing scientists also influence the way nursing theories are developed. Currently, such philosophical stands as relativism, existentialism, phenomenology, general systems philosophy, and material dialectics are found in nursing theorists' writings. Such orientations direct the theoretical formulations of each theorist toward somewhat different directions in terms of the kinds of phenomena selected for study and the approaches developed for nursing strategies.

These orientations are often held by scientists concurrently with philosophies of scientific inquiry. Empirical positivism, physicalism, rationalism, or logical positivism, for example, are held together with philosophies regarding humanity, life, and the world. These philosophies specifically influence the way scientific knowledge is generated. In nursing, the level of sophistication regarding the philosophy of scientific inquiry has not been high. The number of books and articles espousing specific philosophical approaches is growing, indicating a need for our awareness and examination of philosophical impact on scientific development.

## THEORY DEVELOPMENT

Throughout the book, the level of theory development has been explicitly and implicitly expressed. Major theoretical work in nursing still is at the level of theoretical orientations, consisting of major assumptions about the way essential concepts are identified and developed. Propositions in the theories are seldom stated in predictive terms. In general, nursing's theoretical models are mostly descriptive, with some evidence of developing toward explanatory frameworks.

The testability of theoretical statements in nursing theories tends to be limited because of a deficiency in precise designations of empirical referents in the theories. Axiomatization and formalization of theoretical statements have not been attempted, and may be premature with the current state of affairs. A need exists for extensive conceptual clarification of essential phenomena in nursing in order to develop testable theories.

## THEORY-PRACTICE-RESEARCH LINK

Although there is evidence that suggests the narrowing of gaps among these three sectors of the nursing knowledge system, real and "artificial" gaps do exist. Real gaps result from the lack of dialogue among the practitioners of the three areas and from the structural arrangement that segregates practitioners into different organizational settings.

Artificial gaps are the artifacts of discontent, power struggles, and competition among the practitioners in the three functional roles, which result in mutual accusations. In the previous decade, concerns of the profession focused on economic security, public image, and recognition. The profession may have to emerge into a new spirit of scientism in the coming decade. Attempts such as the Rush model, which incorporates three functional areas (teaching, research, and practice) into one nursing role, may be one way of solving the problems of gaps.

Indeed, it is through a close scrutiny of theory in practice and research that nursing can evolve into a viable science, and it is by grounding theoretical formulations in practice and aligning practice problems for research that nursing can expand its scientific richness. Such close scrutiny is needed in order to overcome the real gaps among these three sectors.

## METHODOLOGY

It is an attractive idea to be highly competent in one or two methodologies of scientific inquiry. However, a growing scientific discipline needs to be diverse in its use of techniques of inquiry. The theme for nursing science has to be "discovery" and "expansion." The diversity of subject matter for nursing science necessitates the application of various techniques and methodologies of inquiry and scientific study. Nursing inquiries should test the applicability and limitations of both inductive and deductive methods, and the appropriateness and fidelity of both quantitative and qualitative techniques of research.

## FINAL REMARKS

My exposition in this book has focused on the nature of theoretical thinking rather than on the substance of theories. Since I believe that systematic formulation and reformulation are necessary in nursing for identifying the subject matter and developing theories, I have suggested several different ways of viewing aspects of the world that are of interest to nursing. I have not attempted to evaluate or criticize theories in a systematic or comprehensive manner. I have included in the book those appropriate aspects of nursing and other theories mainly for the purpose of illustration, expansion, and application of ideas under discussion. As suggested in Chapter 1, both theories of nursing and theories in nursing need to be developed, tested, and refined in order to develop a codified body of scientific knowledge that is ultimately required for responsible practice of nursing.

## BIBLIOGRAPHY

Blalock, HM, Jr. *Theory Construction: From Verbal to Mathematical Formulations.* Englewood Cliffs, NJ: Prentice-Hall, 1969

Blalock, HM, Jr. Measurement and Conceptualization Problems: The Major Obstacles to Integrating Theory and Research. *Am Sociol Rev* 44: 881–894, 1979

Carper, B. Fundamental Patterns of Knowing in Nursing. *Adv Nurs Sci* 1, no. 1: 13–23, 1978

Cummings, MK, Becker MH, and Maile, MC. Bringing the Models Together: An Empirical Approach to Combining Variables Used to Explain Health Actions. *J Behav Med* 3: 123–145, 1980

Dickoff, J, and James, P. Theory Development in Nursing. In PJ Verhonick (ed.): *Nursing Research I.* Boston: Little, Brown, 1975, pp 45–92

Donaldson, S, and Crowley, D. The Discipline of Nursing. *Nurs Outlook* 26: 113–20, 1978

Dubin, R. *Theory Building,* Revised edition. New York: The Free Press, 1978

Fawcett, J. The "What" of Theory Development. In *Theory Development: What, Why, How.* New York: National League for Nursing, Publication no. 15–1708, 1978a, pp 17–33

Fawcett, J. The Relationship Between Theory and Research: A Double Helix. *Adv Nurs Sci* 1, no. 1: 49–62, 1978b

Flaskerud, JH, and Halloran, EJ. Areas of Agreement in Nursing Theory Development. *Adv Nurs Sci* 3, no. 1: 1–7, 1980

Glaser, B, and Strauss, A. *The Discovery of Grounded Theory.* Chicago: Aldine, 1967

Greene, JA. Science, Nursing, and Nursing Science: A Conceptual Analysis. *Adv Nurs Sci* 2, no. 1: 57–64, 1979

Hardy, ME. Evaluating Nursing Theory. In *Theory Development: What, Why, How.* New York: National League for Nursing, Publication no. 15–1708, 1978, pp 75–86

Hempel, CG. Formulation and Formalization of Scientific Theories: A Summary Abstract. In F Suppe (ed.): *The Structure of Scientific Theories,* Urbana, IL: University of Illinois Press, 1977, pp 244–265

Jacobs, MK, and Huether, SE. Nursing Science: The Theory-Practice Linkage. *Adv Nurs Sci* 1, no. 1: 63–73, 1978

King, IM. The "Why" of Theory Development. In *Theory Development: What, Why, How.* New York: National League for Nursing, Publication no. 15–1708, 1978, pp 11–16

Kuhn, TS. Second Thoughts on Paradigms. In F Suppe (ed.): *The Structure of Scientific Theories.* Urbana, IL: University of Chicago Press, 1977, pp 459–517

Stevens, BJ. *Nursing Theory: Analysis, Application, Evaluation.* Boston: Little, Brown, 1979

Suppe, F. *The Structure of Scientific Theories.* Urbana, IL: University of Chicago Press, 1977

Toulmin, S. *The Philosophy of Science: An Introduction.* London: Hutchinson, 1953

Toulmin, S. *Human Understanding,* Vol 1. Princeton, NJ: Princeton University Press, 1972

Toulmin, S. Postscript: The Structure of Scientific Theories. In F Suppe (ed.): *The Structure of Scientific Theories.* Urbana, IL: University of Chicago Press, 1977, pp 600–614

# Notes

## Notes to Chapter 1

1. There are several books and articles written with these purposes as the primary focuses. See for example, Margaret E. Mardy, "Evaluating Nursing Theory," in *Theory Development: What, Why, How?* (New York: National League for Nursing, 1978), pp. 75–86; The Nursing Theories Conference Group, *Nursing Theories: The Base for Professional Nursing Practice* (Englewood Cliffs, NJ: Prentice-Hall, 1980); and Barbara J. Stevens, *Nursing Theory: Analysis, Application, Evaluation* (Boston: Little, Brown, 1979).

2. Among the many published work for this subject area, the following books may be of help to serious students of theory construction: Carl G. Hempel, *Fundamentals of Concept Formation in Empirical Sciences* (Chicago: The University of Chicago Press, 1952); Karl R. Popper, *The Logic of Scientific Discovery* (New York: Harper and Row, 1959); Abraham Kaplan, *The Conduct of Inquiry* (San Francisco: Chandler Publishing, 1964); Paul Davidson Reynolds, *A Primer in Theory Construction* (Indianapolis: Bobbs-Merrill, 1971); Robert Dubin, *Theory Building,* Revised edition (New York: The Free Press, 1978); Hubert M. Blalock, Jr., *Theory Construction: From Verbal to Mathematical Formulations* (Englewood Cliffs, NJ: Prentice-Hall, 1969); and Frederick Suppe (ed.), *The Structure of Scientific Theories,* Second edition (Urbana, IL: University of Illinois Press, 1977).

## Notes to Chapter 2

1. One comment about the debate that is going on for a differentiation between "absolute" reality and "conscious" reality may be in order. Many philosophers of science have debated over the definition of reality. The history of scientific discovery tells us that

we are ever encountering phenomena that we were unaware of in our past. This suggests that there exists the "absolute" reality to be discovered, to be aware of. A contrasting view to this is the argument that what we cannot perceive to exist is not reality, and that reality is bounded by the consciousness and perceptiveness of humankind at a given time, for what we cannot fathom to exist cannot be real to us. Such arguments are interesting and paradoxical. But for now, let me ask for the readers' indulgence to accept my position for the duration of this book that a reality needs to be conceptualized in the human mind for it to be problematic.

2. For example, cf. Robert Dubin, *Theory Building,* Revised edition (New York: The Free Press, 1978), and Abraham Kaplan, *The Conduct of Inquiry* (San Francisco: Chandler Publishing, 1964).

3. James Dickoff, Patricia James, and E. Wiedenback, "Theory in a Practice Discipline: Part I. Practice Oriented Theory," *Nursing Research* 17 (1968): 415–435.

4. I do not believe it fruitful to debate over what are proper meanings and definitions of these two terms. While there are many different ways and different levels of specificity with which these terms are used in the scientific community as well as in nursing, the distinction proposed here seems the most accepted way of their uses.

5. Sister Callista Roy and Sharon L. Roberts, *Theory Construction in Nursing: An Adaptation Model* (Englewood Cliffs, NJ: Prentice-Hall, 1981), p. 35.

6. This Hofstadter story labeled as "prelude" should be of interest to readers who want to follow the arguments for holism and reductionism. See Douglas R. Hofstadter, *Gödel, Escher, Bach: An Eternal Golden Braid* (New York: Vintage Books, 1979), p. 282.

### Notes to Chapter 3

1. Many details of this scenario were borrowed from Case 28–1980 of the Case Records of MGH as published in the *New England Journal of Medicine* by Pennington and Mark. Many facts were also altered and created. Thus, the total scenario does not depict an actual case. See: James E. Pennington and Eugene J. Mark, "Case-Record of the Massachusetts General Hospital: Case 28–1980—Pneumonia in a 62-year-old Man with Chronic Lymphocytic Leukemia," *New England Journal of Medicine* 303 (1980): 145–152.

### Notes to Chapter 4

1. See: B.F. Skinner, *Science and Human Behavior* (New York: Macmillan, 1953); Clark L. Hull, *Essentials of Behavior* (New Haven: Yale University Press, 1951); Albert Bandura, *Principles of Behavior Modification* (New York: Holt, Rinehart, and Winston, 1969) for psychological orientation; and George C. Homans, *Social Behavior: Its Elementary Forms* (New York: Harcourt and Brace, 1961); and John Kunkel and Richard H. Nagasawa, "A Behavioral Model of Man: Propositions and Implications," *American Sociological Review* 38 (1973): 530–543 for sociological orientation.

2. See: William B. Cannon, *The Wisdom of the Body* (New York: W.W. Norton and Company, 1931); and Hans O. Selye, *The Stress of Life* (New York: McGraw-Hill, 1956).

3. Herbert Simon, *Models of Thoughts* (New Haven: Yale University Press, 1979), p. 4.

4. For the similarities and differences among the psychoanalytic human models, see the following: Norman O. Brown, *Life Against Death: The Psychoanalytical Meaning of History* (Wesleyan: Wesleyan University Press, 1959); Theodosius Dobzhansky, *The Biology of Ultimate Concern* (New York: The New American Library, 1967); Erik H. Erikson, *Identity and the Life Cycle: Selected Papers* (New York: International Universities Press, 1959); Erik Erikson, *Insight and Responsibility: Lectures on the Ethical Implications of Psychoanalytic Insight* (New York: W.W. Norton, 1964); Erick Fromm, *The Heart of Man: Its Genius for Good and Evil* (New York: Harper and Row, 1964); Erick Fromm and Ramon Xirau (eds.), *The Nature of Man: A Reader* (New York: Macmillan, 1968); Heinz Hartman, *Ego Psychology and the Problems of Adaptation,* Trans. by David Rapoport (New York: International Universities Press, 1958); Philip Rieff, *Freud: The Mind of the Moralist* (New York: Doubleday, 1961); Philip Rieff, *The Triumph of the Therapeutics: The Uses of Faith after Freud* (New York: Harper and Row, 1966); and Don S. Browning, *Generative Man: Psychoanalytic Perspectives* (Philadelphia: The Westminster Press, 1973).

5. In 1970, Rogers proposed four principles of homeodynamics as reciprocity, synchrony, helicy, and resonancy. These were later revised to three principles of homeodynamics as helicy, resonancy, and complementarity. Cf. Martha E. Rogers, *An Introduction to the Theoretical Basis of Nursing* (Philadelphia: F.A. Davis, 1970), and Martha E. Rogers, "Nursing: A Science of Unitary Man," in Joan P. Riehl and Sister Callista Roy, *Conceptual Models for Nursing Practice* (New York: Appleton-Century-Crofts, 1980), pp. 329–337.

6. Although Roy's adaptation model has been said to be based on Helson's adaptation level theory, Roy takes large leaps from Helson's ideas in arriving at her conceptualization. Helson's adaptation level theory is a theory of perceptual adaptation in which perceptual learning is the major theoretical interest. Although Helson alludes to the possibility of expanding his theory to explain other human phenomena, the applicability of the major propositions has not been specified for such an expansion.

7. Andrew C. Twaddle, "The Concept of Health Status," *Social Science and Medicine* 8 (1974): 83.

8. Dorothea E. Orem, *Nursing Concepts of Practice,* Second edition. (New York: McGraw-Hill, 1980), p. 119.

9. Margaret A. Newman, *Theory Development in Nursing* (Philadelphia: F.A. Davis, 1979), pp. 56–58.

10. Index Medicus classifies restlessness as psychomotor agitation, and both terms seem to refer to the same kind of phenomena.

11. Catherine M. Norris, "Restlessness: A Nursing Phenomena in Search of Meaning," *Nursing Outlook* 23 (1975): 104.

### Notes to Chapter 5

1. James K. Feibleman, "The Artificial Environment." In J. Lenihan and W. Fletcher (eds.), *The Built Environment: Environment and Man,* Vol. 8. (New York: Academic Press, 1978), p. 161.

2. Rene Dubos, *Man Adapting* (New Haven: Yale University Press, 1965), p. xvii.

3. Rene Dubos, *Man Adapting* (New Haven: Yale University Press, 1965), p. 261.

4. H.P. Dreitzel (ed.), *The Social Organization of Health* (New York: Macmillan, 1971), p. 3.

5. Emile Durkheim, *Suicide: A Study in Sociology,* Trans. by J.A. Spaulding, and G. Simpson (New York: The Free Press, 1951), p. 299.

6. See, for example, Alexander Solzhenitsyn's *Cancer Ward* for an illuminating insight into the health-care practices in the Gulag.

7. See, for example, C.I. Cohen and J. Sokolovsky, ''Health Seeking Behavior and Social Network of the Aged in Single-Room Occupancy Hotels,'' *Journal of the American Geriatric Society* 27 (1979): 270–278.

8. Among many research writings on the subject, see: B.H. Kaplan, J.C. Cassel, and Susan Gore, ''Social Support and Health,'' *Medical Care* 15 (1977, Supplement): 47–58; Andrew Dean and N. Lin, ''The Stress Buffering Role of Social Support,'' *Journal of Nervous and Mental Disease* 165 (1977): 403–417; K.N. Walker, A. MacBride, and M.L.S. Vachon, ''Social Support Networks and the Crisis of Bereavement,'' *Social Science and Medicine* 11 (1977): 35–41; and S. Henderson, ''The Social Networks, Social Support, and Neurosis: The Function of Attachment in Adult Life,'' *British Journal of Psychiatry* 13 (1977): 185–191.

9. J.M. LaRocco, J.S. House, and J.R.P. French, Jr., ''Social Support, Occupational Stress, and Health,'' *Journal of Health and Social Behavior* 21 (1980): 202–218; J.H. Liem and R. Liem, ''Social Class and Mental Illness Reconsidered: The Role of Economic Stress and Social Support,'' *Journal of Health and Social Behavior* 19 (1978): 139–156; G.C. Andrews et al., ''Life Events, Stress, Social Support, Coping Style and Risk of Psychological Impairment,'' *Journal of Nervous and Mental Disease* 166 (1978): 307–316; and Sidney Cobb and S.V. Kasl, *Termination: The Consequences of Job Loss,* DHEW (NIOSH) Publication No. 77–224, Cincinnati, Ohio, 1977.

10. Twaddle compiled a set of propositions related to sickness behavior and the sick role. See: Andrew C. Twaddle, *Sickness Behavior and the Sick Role,* Cambridge, Mass.: Schenkman Publishing, 1979, Appendix B, pp. 199–206.

## Notes to Chapter 6

1. These statements have been derived from the pages listed in the following: Sister Callista Roy and Sharon L. Roberts, *Theory Construction in Nursing: An Adaptation Model* (Englewood Cliffs, NJ: Prentice-Hall, 1981): pp. 86–90, 197–200, 214–219, 104–109, 125–129, 149–155, 173–181, 236–243, 257–258, 269–270, and 280–281.

2. There are obviously many inconsistencies in the use of the conceptual scheme, especially in suggesting kinds of nursing interventions for different aspects of adaptation modes in Roy and Roberts' discussions.

3. Dorothy Johnson, ''The Behavioral System Model for Nursing,'' in Joan P. Riehl and Sister Callista Roy (eds.), *Conceptual Models for Nursing Practice* (New York: Appleton-Century-Crofts, 1980), p. 242.

4. See: Sister Callista Roy and Sharon L. Roberts, *Theory Construction in Nursing: An Adaptation Model* (Englewood Cliffs, NJ: Prentice-Hall, 1981), pp. 44–48; Martha E. Rogers, *An Introduction to the Theoretical Basis of Nursing* (Philadelphia, F.A. Davis,

1970), p. 125; Imogene M. King, *A Theory for Nursing: Systems, Concepts, Process* (New York: John Wiley, 1981), pp. 8–10; Dorothea E. Orem, *Nursing: Concepts of Practice,* Second edition (New York: McGraw-Hall, 1980), pp. 200–221; and Dorothy E. Johnson, "The Behavioral System Model for Nursing," in Joan P. Riehl and Sister Callista Roy, (eds.), *Conceptual Models for Nursing Practice,* Second edition (New York: Appleton-Century-Crofts, 1980), pp. 238–249.

5. Sister Callista Roy and Sharon L. Roberts, *Theory Construction in Nursing: An Adaptation Model* (Englewood Cliffs, NJ: Prentice-Hall, 1981), pp. 47–48.

6. Martha E. Rogers, *An Introduction to the Theoretical Basis of Nursing* (Philadelphia: F.A. Davis, 1970), p. 126. Italics are mine.

7. Martha E. Rogers, *An Introduction to the Theoretical Basis of Nursing* (Philadelphia: F.A. Davis, 1970), p. 128. Italics are mine.

8. Mi Ja Kim and Derry A. Moritz (eds.), *Classification of Nursing Diagnoses: Proceedings of the Third and Fourth National Conferences* (New York: McGraw-Hill, 1982), p. 219.

9. Kristine M. Gebbie and Mary A. Lavin, *Proceedings of the First National Conference: Classification of Nursing Diagnoses* (St. Louis: C.V. Mosby, 1975), p. 57.

10. Kristine M. Gebbie and Mary A. Lavin, *Proceedings of the First National Conference: Classification of Nursing Diagnoses* (St. Louis: C.V. Mosby, 1975), p. 1.

11. Sister Callista Roy, "A Diagnostic Classification System for Nursing," *Nursing Outlook* 23 (1975): 90.

### Notes to Chapter 7

1. My review for this summarized look was neither systematic nor comprehensive. I believe that a review of selected theoretical books on nursing theories and of three leading scholarly journals in nursing, namely, *Nursing Research, Research in Nursing and Health,* and *Advances in Nursing Science,* covering the period for 1978 through 1981 provided a sufficient base for my purpose. This review is mainly used to indicate the kinds of theoretical and empirical questions that are being raised by nursing scientists currently. I am aware that there are many other journals in which articles dealing with nursing-related phenomena are published. I chose these three journals only because they are nursing oriented and research and or theory oriented.

2. Sister Callista Roy and Sharon L. Roberts, *Theory Construction in Nursing: An Adaptation Model* (Englewood Cliffs, NJ: Prentice-Hall, 1981), p. 62.

# Index